W0018549

CONTROVERSIES IN SCHIZOPHRENIA

Examining timely debates around contentious topics in schizophrenia, *Controversies in Schizophrenia* demonstrates that while some criticisms of psychiatry are pertinent, many are flawed.

Drawing on diverse sources including personal accounts of people with schizophrenia, reports, and psychiatric guidance, this book conceptualises schizophrenia in the context of other psychotic disorders, in order that the condition may be understood better. Key topics covered include antipsychotic medication, a biopsychosocial view, stigma, implications of schizophrenia as an illness, brain anomalies, and neurochemical factors.

This book is essential for mental health professionals working regularly with people with psychosis, including psychiatrists, psychiatric residents, psychologists, nurses, and social workers.

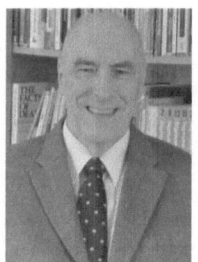 **Michael Farrell** managed a UK-wide psychometric project for City University, London and directed a national initial teacher-training project for the UK Government Department of Education; for over a decade, he led teams inspecting mainstream and special schools and units (boarding, day, hospital, psychiatric). Currently, he works as a private consultant with a range of clients and has lectured and provided consultancy services worldwide.

CONTROVERSIES IN SCHIZOPHRENIA

Issues, Causes, and Treatment

Michael Farrell

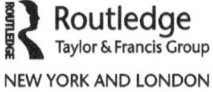

Routledge
Taylor & Francis Group

NEW YORK AND LONDON

Designed cover image: © Getty Images

First published 2024
by Routledge
605 Third Avenue, New York, NY 10158

and by Routledge
4 Park Square, Milton Park, Abingdon, Oxon, OX14 4RN

Routledge is an imprint of the Taylor & Francis Group, an informa business

© 2024 Michael Farrell

ISBN: 978-1-032-53780-1 (hbk)
ISBN: 978-1-032-53779-5 (pbk)
ISBN: 978-1-003-41355-4 (ebk)

DOI: 10.4324/9781003413554

Typeset in Sabon
by MPS Limited, Dehradun

CONTENTS

1

INTRODUCTION

Introduction to the chapter

In this chapter, I introduce basic information on schizophrenia, laying foundations for discussions in the remainder of the volume. This initial information reflects an 'orthodox' psychiatric perspective. In later chapters, this perspective is considered in relation to various topics, and criticisms of it are presented representing a 'dissenting' position.

Turning to the detail of this chapter, I firstly present the personal experiences of schizophrenia of David Boyles and Elyn Saks. Examining how the disorder is currently defined, I look at diagnostic criteria, mainly citing the *DSM-5* (American Psychiatric Association, 2013). From *DSM-5*, I describe the five features of psychosis (like delusions and hallucinations) and other diagnostic requirements. The chapter discusses how early-stage schizophrenia can evade recognition.

Schizophrenia spectrum disorders and other psychotic disorders are examined, for example, delusional disorder, catatonia, brief psychotic disorder, and schizophrenia itself. The chapter explains how, in some mental disorders like schizophrenia, psychosis is 'integral' while in others such as bipolar disorder, it is 'associated.' I look at challenges that arise in delineating schizophrenia, psychosis, and bipolar disorder. The *ICD-11* (World Health Organisation, 2022) its relationship to *DSM-5* is briefly described.

Having laid these foundations, I describe the broad distinction of 'orthodox' and 'dissenting' views of schizophrenia used throughout the present volume. After listing the book's contents, I identify its aims and

DOI: 10.4324/9781003413554-1

distinctive features, and specify intended readers. Finally, the structure of the various chapters is explained, and their contents are set out.

Voices of schizophrenia

David Boyles

David Boyles's (2004) memoir covers several weeks of experiencing psychosis before admission to hospital, his stay in hospital, and events afterwards. Living in St. Augustine, Florida, David has intense feelings of euphoria, and begins to avidly read the Bible, and watch religious television channels. Laid off from work, and with 'psychosis setting in' (Ibid., p. 11) he visits his brother at Virginia Beach. Feeling guilty for reading the Bible and questioning God, David cries increasingly, becoming 'very emotional' (p. 16). His thoughts race. In his bedroom, he sees, 'white figure formations' and 'colourful patterns' (p. 18).

Visiting his parents in New York, David is feels compelled to 'bless the house' (Boyles, 2004, p. 24). He feels God is punishing him. Concerned, his family take him to the local emergency room. Admitted to hospital, and visited by his mother, he hears voices telling him not to scare her (Ibid., p. 31). After a few weeks on medication, he is discharged and returns to Florida, later visiting his brother's Virginia Beach house. There he experiences intrusive thoughts ('non-stop thinking') (p. 41). Included in his hallucinations is, 'a small face looking at me, slowly moving round the edge of the pillows of the couch' (p. 50). Back at work, David attends a support group, taking his medication intermittently. Getting 'shivery sensations' in his head convinces him to take medication regularly (pp. 51–52). Later David starts a new job and attends the community mental health clinic to help him manage his medication. Over Christmas 2002, David experiences 'paranoia' believing that God was punishing him for his being involved in a prank (pp. 59–60).

For David, early warning signs of schizophrenia were: 'hearing and seeing things that aren't there' and making 'irrational statements.' He was unable to sleep, felt that the fundamentals of his personality had changed, and was hyperactive and unable to concentrate. Also, he experienced a high degree of preoccupation with religion, indifference, and 'unusual sensitivity' to sound, light, colour, and textures. He found himself unable to express joy and cried a great deal. David feels that he has accepted his condition and is fortunate in having medication that works for him (pp. 75–76). Explaining his psychosis, he considered that his brain chemistry 'malfunctioned' which brought about thoughts that were not his own and that were 'not valid.' For him, therapy and medication worked together. David states, 'This condition is a biological-chemical imbalance in the brain. **I felt it so I know'** (p. 81, bold in original). His medication helped David to distinguish between reality and delusion. At the time of completing his book, David was living independently and had a new job as an electrical installer (Ibid.).

Elyn Saks

Elyn Saks (2008), professor of law and psychiatry at the University of California, tells of living with schizophrenia. Her experiences as a young student and her later life are recounted as well as the thoughts, feelings, and behaviours associated with her schizophrenia.

At Oxford University, she harbours thoughts of suicide. She thought that she should pour petrol over herself and light a match, which she considered a suitable death for a person as evil as she (Ibid., p. 61). In hospital, meeting with a group of doctors, she is asked why she is not eating and replies in logical, legalistic language presaging her later career. 'Food is evil ... I am evil too, and food would only nourish me. Does it make any sense to you to nourish evil? No, it does not' (p. 74).

Elyn began to feel that she was receiving commands to do things from 'shapeless, powerful beings' that controlled, not with voices, but with thoughts that had been inserted into her head (p. 79). Commands included 'Now lie down and don't move'; 'you are evil' and messages to hurt herself leading her to burn herself with cigarettes, lighters, and electric heaters, and scald herself with boiling water. She states that with psychosis, the division between fantasy and reality are no longer apparent and 'The images I saw, the actions I took were all real, and it made me frantic' (p. 104). One of the worst aspects of schizophrenia was the deep sense of isolation. There is constant awareness that you no longer human, but 'some sort of alien' (p. 179).

Treatments were not always benign. Elyn says that she wrote about these because she had experienced psychosis and knew what it was like. She also knew how metal patients are treated under the law. She speaks of 'the degradation of being tied to a bed against your will and force-fed medicine you didn't ask for.' She desires to see change and wants to bring hope to people with schizophrenia and to bring understanding to others (p. 306).

We now turn to formal definitions and diagnostic criteria for schizophrenia.

Schizophrenia: definitions and diagnostic criteria, and early stages of the disorder

Definition and diagnostic criteria

Briefly, schizophrenia is defined as, 'a serious mental illness that affects how a person thinks, feels, and behaves' and in which individuals may feel that they have, 'lost touch with reality' (National Institute of Mental Health, accessed January 2022).

Further, schizophrenia is 'a serious mental disorder in which people interpret reality abnormally.' It may involve in various combinations, 'hallucinations, delusions, and extremely disordered thinking and behaviour.' These hinder day to day functioning and can be disabling (Mayo Clinic, 2023).

DSM-5 (American Psychiatric Association, 2013) provides diagnostic criteria for schizophrenia. Criterion A specifies five features of psychosis:

- delusions
- hallucinations
- disorganised speech
- grossly disorganised or catatonic behaviour, and
- negative symptoms.

Two or more must be present for a 'significant period' during a month (less if the condition is successfully treated). At least one of the features must be delusions, hallucinations, or disorganised speech (Ibid., p. 99).

Delusions (rigid beliefs, unchanged by conflicting evidence) are often persecutory involving belief that one will be harmed or harassed by another person or organisation. Other typical delusions are referential, grandiose, bizarre (thought withdrawal, thought insertion), and concerning (American Psychiatric Association, 2013, p. 87, paraphrased).

Involuntary 'perception-like experiences' occurring without external stimuli and having the full force of reality typify *hallucinations*. In schizophrenia, the most usual are auditory, often voices (familiar or unfamiliar) that seem 'distinct from' the individuals' own thoughts (Ibid., p. 87).

Someone with *disorganised speech* (indicating disorganised thinking) may switch between topics or respond to questions in a partially related or unrelated way, substantially impairing communication (Ibid., p. 88).

Included in, *grossly disorganised or abnormal motor behaviour* are 'unpredictable agitation' and problems performing goal directed actions. While 'catatonic behaviour' involves a significant decrease in reactions to surroundings like assuming a rigid pose maintained for long periods, 'catatonic excitement' expresses excessive apparently causeless motor activity (Ibid.).

Negative symptoms include reduction in emotional expression, motivated self-initiated purposeful activities, speech output, and capacity for pleasure from positive experiences (Ibid.).

A requirement of criterion B for schizophrenia is that in one or more areas (like work or interpersonal relations), functioning level is markedly below that prior to onset. This occurs for a 'significant portion of time' from the disturbance starting. If the disorder started in childhood or adolescence, there should be evidence of 'failure to achieve expected levels of interpersonal, academic or occupational functioning' (Ibid., p. 87).

Furthermore, 'continuous signs of the disturbance persist for at least six months' (criterion C). Certain disorders have been excluded, namely, schizoaffective disorder and depressive or bipolar disorder with psychotic features (criterion D). The disturbance is not put down to 'the physiological effects of a substance ... or of another medical condition' (criterion E) (Ibid.).

Early stages of schizophrenia

Harder to recognise than the fully developed disorder, early stages of schizophrenia can be camouflaged where indications suggested by various changes are subtle (Torrey, 2019, p. 87–90 and table p. 89).

As observed by the families of individuals who developed schizophrenia, early signs included depression; suspiciousness or feelings that others are talking about one; marked weakness and lack of energy; headaches or strange sensations in the head; confused, strange of bizarre thinking, and social withdrawal (Ibid., p. 89, paraphrased).

Distinguishing schizophrenia within 'schizophrenia spectrum disorders and other psychotic disorders'

It is important is that schizophrenia is distinguished from related conditions. Accordingly, *DSM-5* provides criteria for diagnosing 'schizophrenia spectrum and other psychotic disorders' which of course include schizophrenia itself (American Psychiatric Association, 2013, pp. 87–122). Among these disorders are

- schizotypal (personality) disorder
- delusional disorder
- catatonia
- brief psychotic disorder
- schizophreniform disorder
- substance/medication-induced psychotic disorder
- psychotic disorder due to another medical condition
- schizophrenia, and
- schizoaffective disorder.

Schizotypal personality disorder includes a 'pervasive pattern' of social and interpersonal deficits like lowered capacity for close relationships, distorted cognition or perception, and eccentric behaviour. Although usually beginning in early adulthood, the pattern sometimes occurs earlier. Importantly, 'abnormalities of beliefs, thinking and perception' fall below the threshold at which a psychotic disorder would be diagnosed.

In *delusional disorder* and *catatonia* abnormalities concern only one domain of psychosis. Delusional disorder while involving at least one month of delusions, produces no other psychotic symptoms. Involving decreased motor activity and decreased engagement, or 'excessive and peculiar' motor activity, catatonia is a 'marked psychomotor disturbance' (Ibid., p. 119).

As time-limited conditions, *brief psychotic disorder* lasts more than one day and goes into remission by one month; and *schizophreniform disorder* lasts less than six months, has symptoms like schizophrenia and may not involve functional decline.

Some psychotic disorders are precipitated by another condition. *Substance/medication-induced psychotic disorder* involves psychotic symptoms that are a physiological consequence of a drug of abuse, medication, or exposure to toxins, usually clearing after the implicated agent is removed (Ibid., p. 89). The disorder can be caused by psychoactive substances like alcohol, cannabis, amphetamines, and cocaine; medications such as anaesthetics, analgesics, antidepressants, and anticonvulsants; and toxins like paint. In *psychotic disorder due to another medical condition*, psychotic symptoms are deemed a direct physiological consequence of another medical condition such as cerebral syphilis or multiple sclerosis.

Lasting six months or more, *schizophrenia* includes at least one month of 'active phase symptoms.' As discussed earlier, diagnostic criteria for schizophrenia specify that two or more of the features of psychosis (like delusions and hallucinations) must be present for a 'significant period of time' during a month (Ibid., p. 99).

In *schizoaffective disorder* active phase symptoms of schizophrenia and a mood episode occur together, preceded, or followed by at least two weeks of hallucinations or delusions without prominent mood symptoms (Ibid., p. 89).

Disorders with 'integral' and 'associated' psychosis

In some mental disorders like schizophrenia, psychosis is 'integral.' Psychosis is 'associated' with some other disorders, namely:

- major depressive disorder and persistent depressive disorder (American Psychiatric Association, 2013, pp. 155–188), and
- bipolar disorder which can involve low mood (depression) and elated mood (mania) (Ibid., pp. 123–154).

Depression involves depressed mood and/or faded pleasure in activities that previously have been enjoyed. *Major depressive disorder* can occur with delusions and/or hallucinations (Ibid., p. 162). With 'mood congruent' psychotic features, the content of the hallucinations and delusions reflect depressive themes of 'personal inadequacy, guilt, disease, death, nihilism, or deserved punishment.' Regarding mood incongruent psychotic features, delusions and hallucinations either lack such content or combine mood congruent and incongruent themes (Ibid., p. 186).

Characterised by changes in a person's mood, energy, and functioning ability, *bipolar disorder* involves intense emotional states ('mood episodes') lasting from days to weeks. These are manic/hypomanic (abnormally happy or irritable mood) or depressive (sad mood). Bipolar disorder may occur with 'mood congruent' or 'mood incongruent' psychotic features and with catatonia (American Psychiatric Association, 2013, pp. 127, 132–139).

Challenges in delineating schizophrenia, psychosis, and bipolar disorder

Challenges arise in delineating relationships between schizophrenia and psychosis and relatedly in making distinctions between schizophrenia and bipolar disorder. For example, psychosis, lacks characteristics of a categorical entity. This is reflected by:

- diagnostic problems assessing people jointly presenting symptoms of psychosis and mood,
- high comorbidity between schizophrenia and other mental disorders, and
- difficulties diagnosing sub-threshold psychotic states.

Although schizophrenia is considered categorical, psychotic illness appears more permeating. This suggests caution in having too rigid a separation between mental disorders, and circumspection in using a categorical approach to study psychotic illness (Valle, 2020).

Related to these issues, diagnostically distinguishing schizophrenia from bipolar disorders is, difficult but important regarding, 'therapeutic choices and maintenance programmes' (Altamura et al., 2013, p. 52). Psychosis is noted in 50% or more of patients with bipolar disorder, most often during bipolar mania. Some 48% of manic episodes are accompanied by delusions, 15% by hallucinations, and 19% by formal thought disorder (Ibid.). Indeed, it is debated whether schizophrenia and bipolar disorder are better considered distinct categories of diseases, or as separate dimensions of a single disorder (e.g., Smith, Barch, and Csernansky, 2009).

ICD-11 and its relationship to DSM-5

As well as *DSM-5*, another widely used diagnostic aid is the *International Classification of Diseases and Related Health Problems (ICD-11)* covering similar ground (https://icd.who.int/browse11). *ICD-11* describes and codes 'primary psychotic disorders' encompassing 'schizophrenia and other primary psychotic disorders' characterised by 'significant impairments in reality testing.' The *ICD-11's* categorising of schizophrenia enables diagnosis and clinical management of chronic psychotic conditions. While the *ICD-11* definition of schizophrenia was harmonised with *DSM-5*, differences remain about the duration of symptoms and impaired function (Valle, 2020).

Orthodox and dissenting views

Orthodox position

Underlying debate around schizophrenia are broad perspectives of it. In an 'orthodox' view, schizophrenia is understood within a scientific, medical, and psychiatric framework, and as a biopsychosocial perspective. In this context arise related issues on the course and prognosis of the illness, and treatment including the use of medication and hospitalisation.

An orthodox position recognises categories of mental disorder rather than viewing them as continua associated with relativism. While an orthodox position is biopsychosocial, critics tend to focus on biological aspects of this, claiming that this is the real, underpinning psychiatric view. Orthodox practitioners tend to relate stigma to people's perception of violence associated with schizophrenia.

Orthodoxy recognises genetics, brain morphology, and neurochemistry, as biological aspects of schizophrenia. While appreciating the importance of psychological and social influences, in discussing evidence the focus is often inevitably biological.

Antipsychotic medication is accepted as a useful treatment, while recognising that side effects can be problematic. Antipsychotics are understood in terms of their effect on brain chemistry. Electroconvulsive therapy (ECT) is recognised as an effective treatment in limited instances. Involuntary hospitalisation and treatment are deemed necessary in special circumstances, for example, where a patient endangers themselves or others.

An individual may hold an orthodox position on all the topics touched on, or may have other views of a specific topic, for example, arguing for different causes of stigma. I sometimes use the term, 'orthodox practitioner' to avoid the clumsy phrase, 'person holding an orthodox view.'

Dissenting position

Rejecting that schizophrenia is an illness or disease, a dissenting position adopts a more social and psychological stance. It disavows a biopsychosocial perspective (especially where the focus or topic is perceived as biological) as a medical 'model.' Medical terms like 'treatment' and 'prognosis' and even 'schizophrenia' are avoided or placed in inverted commas to indicate rejection.

Dissenters avoid categorising mental disorders, preferring to see mental disorder and wellness as a continuum. They may take a relativist stance, regarding one theory about schizophrenia as being as justifiable as any other. Seeing orthodoxy as overly biological, a dissenting position valorises psychological and social perspectives. Stigma may be attributed to a fatalistic biological view of schizophrenia.

Because of their biological orientation, genetics, brain anomalies, and neurochemical factors in schizophrenia are viewed suspiciously. Genetics research is regarded as exclusively biological as if its interpretation ignores factors like the environment. Brain anomalies tend to be attributed to causes other than schizophrenia itself, for example to antipsychotic drugs. Neurochemical explanations of schizophrenia are rejected as if they imply that a biological causal factor ties physicians to physical treatment.

Criticising the use of anti-psychotics, and emphasising negative side effects on some patients, dissenters suggest alternatives. ECT is rejected because of perceived risks to life and harmful side effects. Involuntary hospitalisation and treatment are criticised for example for violating patients' rights.

Critics may not cleave to dissenting views in all aspects. For example, they may recognise the usefulness of antipsychotics for some patients. When referring to a person holding a dissenting view, I tend to use expressions like, 'dissenter' or 'critic' rather than the longer clumsier phrase.

Aims and distinctive features of the book and its readers

In presenting topics, this book discusses examples of related evidence and arguments. For instance, in interpreting brain anomalies in schizophrenia, vivid findings are ventricular enlargement and decrease in whole brain volume. Argument centres on whether these are indications of disease or of other factors, like the long-term administration of antipsychotics.

This volume brings together topics generating controversy. In examining the relative positions and how they are presented, I hope that the book will engage people holding different viewpoints. Readers may include mental health professionals, researchers, people with schizophrenia and their families and friends, and others interested in the issues discussed.

Having been fortunate that my previous books have attracted readers in the United States, the United Kingdom, Australia, New Zealand, India, and Southern Africa, I hope that this volume will do the same. It could also be of interest in areas where English, while not the first language, is widely spoken, for example, Scandinavia.

Contents of the book

The chapter titles of this volume reflect some of the main contemporary controversies about schizophrenia, as follows:

1 Introduction
2 Categories, Continua and Relativism
3 A Biopsychosocial Perspective of Schizophrenia
4 Stigma and Schizophrenia
5 Genetics and Schizophrenia
6 Brain Anomalies in Schizophrenia
7 Neurochemical Factors in Schizophrenia
8 Antipsychotics
9 The Continuing Role of Electroconvulsive Therapy
10 Involuntary Hospitalisation and Treatment
11 Challenges and Criticisms
12 Further Criticisms

The chapters form groups as follows:

• Chapters 2 through 4 concern the nature and understanding of schizophrenia
• Chapters 5 through 7 are to do with causes and factors relating to the condition
• Chapters 8 through 10 deal with treatments, and
• Chapters 11 and 12 review types of criticisms that emerged in the book.

Chapter structure

Chapters 2 through 8 have a typical structure. An introduction outlines the chapter contents. The body of the chapter presents several sections concerned with aspects of the topic. A conclusion crystallises some essential points. Further reading is suggested. References are listed at the end of each chapter so that a reader buying a single e-chapter has the requisite citations. We can now consider the contents of each chapter.

Outline of chapters

Chapter 2, '**Categories: Continua and Relativism,**' reiterates the orthodox position that schizophrenia is a category of disorder as reflected in widely used diagnostic guidance. I consider the difficulty of establishing securely the validity and reliability of schizophrenia, and related issues, for example, the challenge of schizophrenia being defined operationally and encroached upon by other conditions. The chapter examines various criticisms and their weaknesses. Criticisms include that schizophrenia was 'invented' by pioneers Kraepelin and Bleuler, and that its conceptualisation lacks scientific rigour. Other criticisms are that a categorical view is based on false assumptions that 'madness' is divisible into a few diseases; and that its symptoms are not understandable via a person's psychology.

Next, I consider alternatives to categorisation proposed by critics, and point to some weakness in these suggestions. One is proposing a continuum extending between wellness and schizophrenia (and psychosis generally) eschewing dividing lines. Another alternative is focusing on symptoms 'within' schizophrenia that tend to occur together. Returning to the orthodox position, I review and endorse arguments for retaining the concept of schizophrenia. This involves recognising justifiable criticism and responding accordingly, while refining the concept according to new evidence.

Chapter 3, '**A Biopsychosocial Perspective of Schizophrenia,**' outlines an orthodox biopsychosocial understanding of schizophrenia which identifies it as a brain disorder understood in medical terms, while taking account of psychological and social factors in both understanding causation, and in treatment. I discuss criticisms that the orthodox approach to schizophrenia emphasises physical aspects which dissenters negatively describe as a 'medical model.'

Accordingly, critics may claim that seeing schizophrenia as a physical illness, assumes that it necessitates a solely physical treatment like medication, or electroconvulsive therapy. Another criticism is that a medical approach is pessimistic about the chances of recovery from schizophrenia, seeing it as an incurable illness. Critics may take a subjectivist view in which there is no external or objective truth. Relatedly, understanding schizophrenia as an illness may be regarded as just another theory. I look at rhetorical devices in criticism such as the use of emotive language. Weaknesses in each of these criticisms are identified.

Chapter 4, '**Stigma and Schizophrenia,**' examines an orthodox view that stigma is associated with the incidence of rare violence perpetrated by people with schizophrenia. I argue that focusing on criminal records underestimates the prevalence of aggressive behaviour, and the burden of coping with schizophrenia experienced by families and professionals.

The chapter considers the negative impact of high-profile acts of violence on public perceptions, and the impact on families and friends of victims killed by individuals with schizophrenia.

In a dissenting view, stigma towards schizophrenia can be created by orthodox psychiatry (depicted as 'biological psychiatry'). Relatedly, I examine critics' mistrust of drug company marketing and research. The chapter considers criticisms that mental health literacy as a destigmatising programme was too biological, becoming an opportunity to educate the public about the biological basis of schizophrenia, and its treatment by medication. I review research reporting associations between causal beliefs of mental disorder (biogenetic or psychosocial) and attitudes or desire for social distance; and consider experimental studies. These link biogenetic causal beliefs with negative attitudes, and psychosocial beliefs with positive attitudes. However, only a few studies relate to schizophrenia, and all concern only projected attitudes, not real-life behaviour.

In Chapter 5, '**Genetics and Schizophrenia**', I summarise an orthodox position. This recognises progress in understanding as contemporary research has replaced earlier notions of single gene causation with a more complex picture. Continuing challenges recognised by orthodox practitioners are considered. One is variability in clinical manifestation of schizophrenia and the absence of a biomarker to compensate for shortcomings in phenotypic demarcation. A response to this draws on endophenotypes. These aim to bridge the gap between high-level symptom presentation and low-level genetic variability, attempting to segment behavioural symptoms into more stable phenotypes with a genetic link.

I consider criticisms each with their own limitations. Some dissenting critics refer potentially misleadingly to a genetic 'basis' of schizophrenia. They may emphasise old studies indicating familial factors while underplaying more 'direct' research like genome-wide association studies (GWAS). Overstatement may be used to bolster a weak position. Critics may choose nebulous targets so individuals and groups are unable to respond, may make unjustifiable generalisations, and may impute malign motivations to genetic researchers evoking Nazi atrocities.

Chapter 6, '**Brain Anomalies and Schizophrenia**,' discusses imaging techniques like computerised tomography (CT) or magnetic resonance imagery (MRI) scans indicating structural and functional anomalies in people with schizophrenia. Among structural deficits are grey matter volume, and the disruption of white matter integrity. Functional anomalies include abnormal neural activity when doing memory tasks. Specific parts of the brain related to changes include lateral ventricle enlargement.

Challenges have been made towards studies of brain differences in people with schizophrenia. It has been argued that large ventricles are not a specific cause of schizophrenia given their appearance in other conditions, like alcoholism. Also, environmental factors like childhood trauma may contribute to the development of schizophrenia and may be associated with brain anomalies. Critics may overstate evidence to argue that antipsychotics cause brain anomalies. They may depict drug funded research findings and associated researchers as ideological, while giving a laudatory presentation of selected supportive evidence. I examine weaknesses in such dissenting views.

Chapter 7, '**Neurochemical Factors in Schizophrenia**,' looks at the different iterations of the dopamine hypothesis. The chapter shows how, as further evidence accumulated about earlier versions, they were modified. The 'original' dopamine hypothesis was that excessively active dopamine transmission leads schizophrenia symptoms. Version 2 pointed to brain areas involving excessive or depleted dopamine transmission. Version 3 offered a framework linking risk factors like stress to increased presynaptic striatal dopaminergic function. Further revisions are envisaged leading to a version 4.

The chapter argues that some dissenting views are flawed. For example, the idea that the original dopamine hypothesis is still current and 'popular' overlooks extensive work on developments of the hypothesis. Criticism that the original dopamine theory is simplistic and unsubstantiated is outdated, as the hypothesis has developed. Claiming that researchers have continually failed to confirm the dopamine ('lead') hypothesis misunderstands that hypotheses must be refutable and modifiable leading to better versions.

Chapter 8, '**Antipsychotics**,' looks at the fortuitous development of chlorpromazine, the first antipsychotic drug. Next it outlines some types of antipsychotics and their efficacy, looking at first- and second-generation antipsychotics. The chapter discusses various adverse side effects of sedation, weight gain, adverse sexual outcomes, and movement disorders.

I look at criticisms of the use of antipsychotics and at some weakness of these views. For example, dissenting voices may emphasise adverse effects of medication rather than how to avoid them, such as by differentiating between the risks associated with different antipsychotics. The chapter considers the view that claims associated with some pharmaceutical companies invite caution. For example, accusations are made of pharmaceutical firms distorting the reporting of drug benefits. Proposals that may alleviate such concerns are touched on.

In Chapter 9, '**The Continuing Role of Electroconvulsive Therapy**,' I illustrate polarised personal accounts of ECT as well as current (more consistently positive) patient perspectives. I describe modern procedures for administering ECT. The chapter outlines theories about how ECT works. I mention conditions treated with ECT including its occasional use with schizophrenia and cite recent studies showing the positive effects of the therapy.

Criticisms of ECT are discussed. For example, regarding efficacy, I examine critics' negative and emotive colouring of descriptions of pioneering work. I suggest that critics underestimate limitations of earlier studies showing weak ECT efficacy. Risks of ECT are discussed, including of memory impairment. I note that despite critics' reference to older research, current evaluations find no evidence that mortality associated with ECT exceeds that of minor procedures using general anaesthetics. Also, discussing ECT and brain damage, critics may interpret research pessimistically, while current UK guidance cites studies showing no evidence that ECT causes brain damage.

Chapter 10, 'Involuntary Hospitalisation and Treatment,' examines the aims of hospitalisation like allowing observation and assessment of patients in a controlled setting, and providing respite for families. I look at alternatives such as coordinated specialty care programmes. The chapter considers rehabilitation to reduce rehospitalisation, for instance community 'clubhouses' for people having had mental disorders. Therapeutic community alternatives for people with schizophrenia are discussed. Legal US state underpinnings of involuntary commitment of patients to psychiatric settings are outlined. I consider reasons for hospitalisation and physical restraint.

The chapter discusses the 1987 UN *Convention against Torture and Other Cruel, Inhuman or Degrading Treatment or Punishment* and the 2012 UN *Convention on the Rights of Persons with Disabilities*. I consider Méndez' (2013) report as a UN rapporteur which draws on the two UN Conventions and links some psychiatric provision and treatments; to torture and related treatment or punishment. The chapter discusses a report of the Center for Human Rights and Humanitarian Law: Anti-Torture Initiative (2013) comprehensively rebutting Méndez' proposals. I propose that there remains a strong case for involuntary hospitalisation and treatment in specified circumstances.

In Chapter 11, 'Challenges and Criticisms,' draws together points arising in previous chapters. I briefly reiterate some examples of the challenges relating to schizophrenia like schizophrenia's weak validity and reliability, and the permeability of psychosis. After this, I review types of dissenting criticisms of schizophrenia, pointing out their weaknesses. I first cover overstatement, emotive language, euphemism, and other rhetorical devices. For example, instances of overstatement include criticism that schizophrenia is unscientific paralleling astrology, and an overly negative depiction of genetic research.

Another type of dissenting criticism identified by the chapter concerns conflicting and weak evidence. Examples are criticisms that the 'medical model' is pessimistic and proposing that understanding schizophrenia as an illness is just another theory.

Chapter 12, '**Further Criticisms**,' examines further dissenting views of research into schizophrenia and understanding of the disorder. I point out the weaknesses of these criticisms. The chapter discusses distorting emphases, illogical criticisms and positions, misrepresenting biopsychosocial psychiatry as purely biological, focusing on old research or old versions of a theory or explanation, the use of a distorted redefinition of 'torture,' and other topics.

For example, regarding distorting emphases, the chapter considers disputable emphases when reviewing genetic research, and criticism putting the spotlight on adverse effects of antipsychotics rather how to reduce or avoid side effects. Also discussed are dissenters' views of ECT related deaths which may place a misleading emphasis on older research, and critics emphasising the simplistic, outdated, reductionist, unsubstantiated, contextless, and crude.

References

Altamura, C. A., Dragogna, F., Pozzoli, S. and Mauri, M. C. (2013) 'Schizophrenia: Differential diagnosis and comorbidities' in Kasper, S. and Papadimitriou, G. N. (Eds.) (2nd Edition) *Schizophrenia: Biopsychosocial Approaches and Current Challenges* (Medical Psychiatry Series). New York and London, Informa Healthcare (pp. 52–69).

American Psychiatric Association (2013) *Diagnostic and Statistical Manual of Mental Disorders Fifth Edition (DSM5)*. Washington DC, APA.

Boyles, D. (2004) *My Punished Mind: A Memoir of Psychosis*. New York, iUniverse.

Center for Human Rights and Humanitarian Law: Anti-Torture Initiative (2013) *Torture in Healthcare Settings: Reflections on the Special Report on Torture's 2013 Thematic Report*. American University Washington College of Law - Center for Human Rights and Humanitarian Law (December 2013).

Mayo Clinic (2023) 'Schizophrenia' (accessed January 2023). https://www.mayoclinic. org/diseases-conditions/schizophrenia/symptoms-causes/syc-20354443

Méndez, J. E. (2013) *Report of the Special Rapporteur on Torture and Other Cruel, Inhuman or Degrading Treatment or Punishment*. New York, United Nations, Human Rights Council. http://www.hr-dp.org/files/2013/ 10/28/A. HRC.22.53SpecialRappReport.2013.pdf

National Institute of Mental Health (accessed 2022) *Assertive Community Treatment*. https://www.nimh.nih.gov/

Saks, E. R. (2008) *The Centre Cannot Hold: My Journey Through Madness*. New York, Virago.

Smith, M. J., Barch, D. M. and Csernansky, J. G. (2009) 'Bridging the gap between schizophrenia and psychotic mood disorders: Relating neurocognitive deficits to psychopathology' *Schizophrenia Research* 107, 1, 69–75.

Torrey, E. F. (2019) (7th Edition) *Surviving Schizophrenia: A Family Manual.* New York and London, Harper Perennial.

United Nations (1984) *Convention against Torture and Other Cruel, Inhuman or Degrading Treatment or Punishment.* United Nations (came into force in 1987).

United Nations (2012) *Convention on the Rights of Persons with Disabilities.* United Nations.

Valle, R. (2020) 'Schizophrenia in ICD-11: Comparison of ICD-10 and DSM-5' *Journal of Psychiatry and Mental Health* 13, 2, 95–104 April-June 2020 (translated from the Spanish). https://www.elsevier.es/en-revista-revista-psiquiatria-salud-mental-486-articulo-schizophrenia-in-icd-11-comparison-icd-10-S2173505020300145

World Health Organisation (2022) *International Classification of Diseases and Related Health Problems (ICD-11).* World Health Organisation. https://www.who.int/standards/ classifications/classification-of-diseases

2
CATEGORIES, CONTINUA AND RELATIVISM

Introduction

In this chapter, I briefly reiterate the orthodox position that schizophrenia is a category of disorder. Taking a similar stance, the *Diagnostic and Statistical Manual of Mental Disorders Fifth Edition (DSM-5)* seeks to distinguish schizophrenia from other disorders. It does this through diagnostic criteria and by identifying differences between disorders like severity and duration. Also conceptualising schizophrenia as a category is the *International Classification of Diseases and Related Health Problems (ICD-11)*.

I consider the difficulty of establishing securely the validity and reliability of schizophrenia, and related issues. These concern the challenges of schizophrenia being defined operationally and being encroached by related conditions; and schizophrenia having no single cause and the different causes not always being present. Also problematic is that schizophrenia is defined by symptoms. This is potentially misleading because different disorders can produce the same symptoms, while no single symptom securely identifies schizophrenia. Furthermore, although schizophrenia is seen as categorical, psychotic illness appears more permeating, which may suggest avoiding too rigid a separation between mental disorders. Implications of these issues are discussed.

The chapter examines the criticism that schizophrenia was 'invented' by psychology founders Kraepelin and Bleuler, a weak argument unhelpfully drawing on emotive language and euphemism (equating schizophrenia with common unusual behaviours). I next discuss the criticism that the conceptualisation of schizophrenia lacks scientific rigour. This presents an

DOI: 10.4324/9781003413554-2

orthodox categorical view as based on false assumptions that madness can be divided into a small number of diseases, and that symptoms of madness cannot be understood in terms of a person's psychology. I argue that these are not assumptions but propositions that can be examined and tested, rendering the criticism overstated and unfounded.

As well as criticising, dissenters have proposed alternatives to categorisation. One is adopting a continuum extending between wellness and schizophrenia (and psychosis more generally) and having no firm dividing lines. However, I argue that symptoms of psychosis are generally different in degree to what most people routinely experience. Suggesting a slight difference between ordinarily hearing voices and psychosis downplays the gulf between them. I discuss another alternative to categorisation – an approach focusing on identifiable symptoms 'within' schizophrenia that tend to occur together. Examples are positive symptoms like hallucinations, and negative symptoms such as reduced emotional expression. This approach, the chapter notes, may be used for assessment and treatment, but its reliability is questioned where clinicians disagree about whether a patient has a particular symptom.

Returning to the orthodox position, I review and endorse arguments for retaining the category of schizophrenia. This involves recognising where criticism is justifiable and responding accordingly, while refining the concept of schizophrenia according to new evidence.

Orthodox and dissenting positions

In an orthodox position, schizophrenia is part of a spectrum of disorders. Some have the 'full-blown' syndrome, while others have a lesser form, like schizotypal personality disorder. Members of the general population may sometimes experience psychotic manifestations like hallucinations, but these are not one end of the 'schizophrenia spectrum.' On the contrary, schizophrenia is seen as a 'categorical brain disease' (Torrey, 2019, p. 63). Lists of symptoms can suggest that schizophrenia may be diagnosed comparatively easily, which in its 'fully developed form' it often is. However, in its early stages, schizophrenia is hard to diagnose with full confidence (Ibid., p. 56). Criteria like *Diagnostic and Statistical Manual of Mental Disorders Fifth Edition (DSM-5)* in its periodically updated iterations, has helped to make the diagnosis of schizophrenia more precise, but 'problems persist.' Diagnosis still involves a psychiatrists' 'evaluation of patients' behaviour' which to some degree is subjective (Ibid., p. 57).

A dissenting view maintains that there is 'widespread confusion' about the term schizophrenia relating to its 'meaning, boundaries and even value' (Murray and Dean, 2008, p. 285). Kraepelin and Bleuler, two founders of modern psychiatry, are said to be responsible for the 'invention' of schizo-phrenia. This represents a continuation of a 'futile search for categories of unusual behaviours' in the expectation of finding illnesses. The 'invention' also continues past themes of 'social control and harmful treatments' which are concealed by theories about help for 'defective individuals' (Read, 2013a, p. 20). Schizotypy assists in understanding the 'aetiology, develop-ment, and expression of schizophrenia-spectrum psychopathology.' It offers a construct to bring together a 'continuum of clinical and subclinical manifestations' (Kwapil and Barrantes-Vidal, 2015, p. S366 abstract). It is claimed taking such a continuum view that many people sometimes hear voices or have fears or beliefs that are not shared by other people. If stress is high enough, for anyone, such experiences could, 'shade into psychosis' (Cooke, 2017, p. 113, section 14.1).

Schizophrenia as a category of disorder: a preamble

In the previous chapter, I outlined definitions of schizophrenia and related matters. Schizophrenia was, 'a serious mental illness that affects how a person thinks, feels and behaves' and in which individuals may feel they, '... have lost touch with reality' (National Institute for Mental Health, accessed 2022). The earlier chapter described criteria for identifying schizophrenia used in *DSM-5* (American Psychiatric Association, 2013). *DSM-5* diag-nostic criteria for schizophrenia included reference to five features of psy-chosis (delusions, hallucinations, disorganised speech, grossly disorganised or catatonic behaviour, and negative symptoms) (Ibid., p. 99), and the duration and impact of the condition (American Psychiatric Association, 2013, p. 87).

I outlined *DSM-5* guidance for following a sequence of diagnosing and differentiating schizophrenia spectrum disorders and other psychotic dis-orders (American Psychiatric Association, 2013, pp. 87–122). Schizophrenia spectrum disorders ranged from schizotypal (personality) disorder to 'unspecified schizophrenia spectrum and other psychotic disorder' and of course included schizophrenia itself. Schizophrenia (in which psychosis is integral) is distinguished from other disorders in which psychosis is associ-ated, namely major depressive disorder and persistent depressive disorder, and bipolar disorder. Diagnostically differentiating schizophrenia from bipolar disorders is especially problematic.

In all this, *DSM-5* takes a categorical approach, while seeking to carefully distinguish schizophrenia from other disorders. It does this through pro-viding diagnostic criteria and by identifying differences between the various disorders like severity and duration. Similarly, the *ICD-11* (World Health Organisation, 2021) conceptualises schizophrenia from a categorical standpoint. Its definition of schizophrenia was harmonised with *DSM-5* with the removal of first-rank symptoms, although differences remain about the duration of symptoms and impaired function (Valle, 2020).

Having briefly reiterated the conceptualisation of schizophrenia as a category, we can now look at challenges that it poses, beginning with difficulties arising from categorisation in general and moving on to challenges facing schizophrenia specifically.

Challenges: schizophrenia's weak validity and reliability; and the permeability of psychosis

Validity and reliability; and the permeability of psychosis

Broad criticisms are made about categories of mental disorder. Rutter (2013) maintains that there are too many categories in *DSM-5* 'for any clinician to remember the criteria for each.' Furthermore, the co-occurrence of diagnoses is 'unacceptably high.' Rutter argues that 'growing evidence' of a lack of distinctiveness between some diagnoses is ignored. Also, while future research findings pertinent to classifications might lead to 'modifications in the classification,' it is unclear who will decide when this is necessary and how it will be done.

Another challenge concerns the risks of restrictive labelling and stigma. It is that classification can come to define someone exclusively as if they were no more in total than the classification. A person with symptoms of a mental disorder can be seen as 'a schizophrenic' or 'a depressive' and nothing else. Ignored is their role as a parent, an employee or employer, a sports enthusiast, a student, and so on. In other words, a category can become a restricting label. In attempts to avoid this, others sometimes refer to the person first, being careful to speak of 'a person with schizophrenia' or 'a person with psychotic disorder.'

More specific to schizophrenia, critics maintain that the category is neither valid enough nor sufficiently reliable to ensure secure identification (Bentall, 2003, pp. 44–47). Stefanis and Stefanis (2009) state that a central difficulty is that it schizophrenia, 'is defined operationally, is encroached by neighbouring entities, and still lacks identity validation' (Ibid., p. 1).

Unlike many physical illnesses with a determinable cause that can help to confirm the existence of the disease, schizophrenia lacks a single origin. Many possible causal indications exist, for example relating to brain structure and functioning, but these are not always present. Psychotic disorders like schizophrenia are defined by their symptoms, which may mislead because different disorders can produce the same symptoms. Also, no single symptom definitively identifies schizophrenia.

In practice, symptoms may be evasive because the person being assessed tries to conceal them, or because schizophrenia is episodic and is not showing itself at the time of assessment. Diagnosis is dependent upon a psychiatrist's informed but still partly subjective judgement based on what the patient is doing and saying (Torrey, 2019, pp. 66–67). Such subjectivity is helpful in allowing a clinician the flexibility to use professional experience and judgement, but also introduces a further element of variation.

Valle (2020) identifies issues concerning schizophrenia as a category arising in *ICD-11*. These concern the extent to which the conditions of psychosis, included under the construct of schizophrenia, lack characteristics of a categorical entity. This is reflected by diagnostic problems when assessing cases jointly presenting symptoms of psychosis and mood, high comorbidity presented by schizophrenia with other mental disorders, and difficulties in the diagnosis of sub-threshold psychotic states.

Consequently, although schizophrenia is seen as categorical, psychotic illness appears more permeating. This suggests not trying to separate mental disorders in too rigid a fashion, and questioning the suitability of a categorical approach for studying psychotic illness (Ibid.).

Implications and responses

Among implications of challenges to improving the reliability and validity of the construct of schizophrenia, already touched on is that it can make diagnosis and interpretations of research findings more difficult. Related to this is the consistency of recommendations in practice guidelines in different countries. Differences exist between in Britain, the National Institute for Care and Health Excellence (NICE) guidelines for schizophrenia (NICE, 2014) and the recommendations of the US Schizophrenia Patient Outcomes Research Team (PORT) (Hogan, 2010; Kreyenbuhl et al., 2010). For example, social skills training is recommended by PORT but not by NICE.

Contributing to these differences may be different methods of reviewing the literature informing the guidelines, but underlying this is likely issues of reliability and validity already discussed. One result is reduced clarity about what does and does not work, muddying the waters of empirical literature for clinicians and potentially detracting from implementing supported interventions.

Challenges concerning the validity and reliability of schizophrenia and the permeability of psychosis raise a key choice. Do clinicians, researchers, and others abandon the construct of schizophrenia, or do they develop and refine it based on existing and emerging evidence? Dissenters tend to favour the first option, while orthodox practitioners are inclined to support the second. Towards the end of the current chapter, this important issue will be revisited.

Criticism that schizophrenia was invented – euphemism and emotive language

Read (2013a) in a book chapter titled 'The invention of "schizophrenia": Kraepelin and Bleuler' claims that Emile Kraepelin and Eugene Bleuler, two founders of modern psychiatry were responsible for the invention of schizophrenia. What might such a claim mean?

'Invention' can convey the action of innovating something, perhaps developing a process such as smelting iron, or creating equipment like a sewing machine. Also, the term can indicate making something up or expressing a piece of fantasy as when someone invents a false alibi, presenting it as true. Reid evidently intends the second meaning of invention. Yet he fails to convincingly convey why early attempts to understand and define behaviour described as schizophrenia should persuade the two founders to invent untrue observations and explanations.

But Read (2013a) further maintains that the invention of schizophrenia 'represents a continuation of the futile search for categories of unusual behaviours in the hope of discovering illnesses' (Ibid.). This suggests schizophrenia is no more than unusual behaviours which would equate symptoms like life impairing catatonic states with speaking too loudly. It also implies that malevolence guides anyone who would interpret unusual behaviour as an illness. Euphemising disturbing and potentially harmful behaviour associated with schizophrenia as simply 'unusual' allows Read to castigate those who see it as an illness.

Read (2013a) also claims that the invention of schizophrenia represents a further step in 'the historical themes of social control and harmful treatments disguised by theories about help for defective individuals' (Ibid.). This neo-Marxist Foucauldian posture in which harmful treatments are nurtured by structurally oppressive society surely misrepresents the work of the early pioneers and the perspectives of modern psychiatry.

In describing early developments, Read (2013a, p. 32) states that psychiatry survived its crisis, but at 'an appalling cost for the millions who for a century thereafter have been branded with the scientifically meaningless and socially devastating label "schizophrenia"' (Ibid.). The idea of being branded like an animal and at the same time being scarred by the experience shifts rational comment into emotive rhetoric.

Criticism that schizophrenia is unscientific paralleling astrology – overstatement

Bentall (2003) maintains that an 'orthodox position' rests on two incorrect 'assumptions.' The first of these is that, 'madness can be divided into a small number of diseases (for example schizophrenia and manic depression).' The second assumption is that, 'manifestations or "symptoms" of madness cannot be understood in terms of the psychology of the person who suffers from them' (Ibid., p. 8). But is an orthodox position based solely on *assumptions*, that is, propositions taken as true without sufficient evidence or proof?

Bentall's (2003) first proposition (that madness is divisible into a few diseases, like schizophrenia) can be, and is, tested as criteria for schizophrenia are developed. Such criteria, coupled with professional judgement, can usefully identify specific disorders. Any weaknesses in such criteria can be, and are, modified and refined. Orthodox practitioners accept there is evidence for schizophrenia as a distinct disorder. Dissenters maintain that disorders including schizophrenia cannot be usefully identified.

What of the second proposition that orthodoxy incorrectly assumes that symptoms of madness cannot be understood within a person's psychology? An orthodox biopsychosocial perspective rejects this accusation, recognising the importance of psychological and social factors. Some dissenters, tending to see orthodox views as purely biological, continue to maintain that orthodoxy ignores personal psychology.

Because these two claims are not assumptions but propositions, each is testable according to evidence. Bentall (2003, p. 155) incorrectly identifies two propositions about schizophrenia as 'assumptions' that ignore rational debate and evidence. Under this misapprehension, he then distorts orthodox psychiatry. For over a century, he maintains, people have harboured 'serious misunderstandings' about madness. Also, 'many contemporary approaches to the problem, although cloaked with the appearance of scientific rigor, have more in common with astrology than rational science.'

But to equate a debate in which evidence is presented and accepted or rejected with astrology is misleading rhetoric, overstating the position. In considering these issues, orthodox psychiatry settles for looking at evidence, not gazing at the stars.

Continua as an alternative to categorisation and its weakness-misleading euphemistic parallels

Dissenters do not only offer criticisms; they also suggest alternatives to categorisation. An example is envisaging mental disorders including schizophrenia as a continuum. Skull (2011) maintains that any seeming boundaries between 'madness and malingering,' and between 'insanity and eccentricity' lack clarity. 'Modern psychiatry,' he believes, tries to 'obfuscate and obscure the existence of continuing profound uncertainties about how to establish the boundaries between the mad and the sane' (Ibid., p. 2). However, this overstates the case.

Because it is not always clear where to set the boundaries of sanity, and there are 'uncertainties' (profound or otherwise), this does not imply that distinctions are not possible. In physical illness, there is not always certainty about separating a real illness and malingering, but this does not imply that the designation of illness be dropped. Skull's (2011) vague personalising of 'modern psychiatry' as trying to 'obscure and obfuscate' evades challenge. Attacking a nebulous entity rather than an individual or group of people, ensures that there is no one to question the position.

Related to the claim of unclear boundaries is the proposal of a continuum. 'Schizotypy' refers to the proposed existence of a continuum of personality characteristics and experiences. These, it is claimed, range from normal dissociative states to extremes related to psychosis and schizophrenia. This contrasts to a categorical view of schizophrenia seen as a pathological state which a person has or does not have.

Certain dissenters propose that a continuum extends between wellness and schizophrenia (and psychosis more generally) having no firm dividing lines. Some individuals experience hallucinations but are not considered to have a mental disorder. Others have weird beliefs like aliens abducting earthlings but are not necessarily considered psychotic. This approach eschews boundaries between mental disorder and mental illness, claims that there are no discrete mental illnesses, and maintains that categorical diagnoses insufficiently define the nature of psychological complaints (Bentall, 2003, p. 143, Table 6.1).

A report, *Understanding Psychosis and Schizophrenia* claims that 'there is no clear dividing line between "psychosis" and other thoughts, feelings and beliefs' (Cooke, 2017, p. 6, Executive Summary). Neither is there a dividing line, between 'psychosis' and 'normality.' Indeed, 'There is no "us" and "them"' (Ibid., p. 113, section 14.1). Some people, the report reiterates, have a traditional perspective of schizophrenia or psychosis as an illness, while others do not. It maintains, that, 'a more helpful and accurate view is probably to see experiences as on a continuum' (Ibid., p. 23).

Cooke (2017) also has related things to say about hearing voices, thought disorder, and delusions. Seemingly, many people experience hearing voices, 'occasionally or to a minor degree, for example at times of stress.' For others, hearing voices is, 'more intense, enduring and/or distressing' (Ibid., p. 17, section 3, key points). Also, many people when stressed can become, 'somewhat "thought disordered" and say confused or confusing things' (Ibid., p. 11, section 1.1). Delusions are seen as 'unusual' beliefs that are 'very similar to other beliefs or prejudices' (Ibid., p. 47, section 7.3). They involve holding convictions not held by others around you for example, 'that there is a conspiracy against you by the CIA, or that someone else is controlling your thoughts' (Ibid., p. 10, section 1.1). If the level of stress is high enough, such experiences could 'shade into psychosis' (Ibid., p. 113, section 14.1). Yet some of these parallels between everyday experiences and schizophrenia and psychosis are misleading. Symptoms of psychosis are generally so different in degree to what most people ordinarily experience that they are effectively different in kind.

Some people may hear voices to a small extent, and for others they can be 'intense, enduring and/or distressing' (Cooke, 2017, p. 17, section 3, key points). But to say that if someone experiences sufficient stress these experiences may 'shade into psychosis' suggests merely a slight distinction between ordinarily hearing voices and psychosis, downplaying their marked differences. It is implied that the thought disorder of psychosis is like getting mixed up when we are 'emotionally stressed' (Ibid., p. 11, section 1.1). Yet in psychiatry, thought disorder involves a level of disorganisation 'so severe as to substantially impair communication' (American Psychiatric Association, 2013, p. 107). Delusions might be equated with cleaving to strong beliefs that 'others around you do not share' (Cooke, 2017, p. 10, section 1.1). But delusions in psychiatry are 'fixed beliefs that are not amenable to change in the light of conflicting evidence' (American Psychiatric Association, 2014, p. 87). Having deeply held political views when in a group adhering to opposing convictions involves 'holding strong beliefs that others around you do not share.' Having a fixed belief that an intelligence agency is conspiring against you is quite different.

Other indications of psychosis are even harder to equate to ordinary experience and behaviour. Catatonia involves assuming a 'rigid posture for long periods' while negative symptoms are characterised by a decline in 'motivated self-initiated purposeful activities' (American Psychiatric Association, 2014, p. 88).

Using syndromes and symptoms not categories in identification and assessment and its weaknesses – conflicting evidence

As another alternative to categorising, some critics who consider schizophrenia too heterogeneous propose identifying cohering groups of symptoms 'within' schizophrenia.

Groups of symptoms

Groupings have included clusters of positive symptoms (like hallucinations and delusions) on the one hand, and clusters of negative symptoms (such as reduced emotional expression) on the other. This indicates that people not having groups of negative symptoms tend to have a better prognosis (Strauss et al., 2010). As well as positive and negative syndromes, a disorganisation syndrome is also cited (Cohen and Docherty, 2005).

Relatedly, Kirkpatrick et al. (2001) propose a focus on clusters of symptoms within schizophrenia in a 'multiple disease' theory. Firstly, they suggest treating schizophrenia itself as a clinical syndrome rather than a single disease. Identifying 'specific diseases within the syndrome' they argue could help in developing more specific treatments. 'Deficit pathology' (enduring, idiopathic negative symptoms), they propose, defines a group different from those with schizophrenia that do not have these deficits. It is maintained that deficit and non-deficit groups differ in 'signs and symptoms, biological correlates, treatment response, and etiological factors' (Ibid., abstract).

Symptoms as the focus of intervention

Reducing the focus further, researchers and clinicians may concentrate on symptoms of schizophrenia like hallucinations for assessment and treatment. Sometimes these symptoms are called 'complaints' to avoid unintended implications of psychiatric conditions. A study by Cohen and Docherty (2005) suggested that the positive syndrome has few clinically significant neuropsychological associates. However, hallucination and delusion *severity scores* when analysed independently were associated with different patterns of neuropsychological functioning. This the authors claim, suggests that a symptom-oriented approach may be more sensitive and informative than a syndrome approach in investigating neuropsychological functioning across the diverse manifestations of schizophrenia.

Criticisms are made of the reliability of a symptoms approach. That is, researchers and clinicians disagree less about whether a patient has a particular symptom than whether they fitted a specified diagnosis (Mojtabai and Rieder, 1998). Bentall (2003, pp. 144–145) argues that some reported measures of reliability of symptoms are likely underestimates of what can be achieved. When assessments have been specially designed to measure specific symptoms, high levels of inter-rater agreement have been found (Carter et al., 1995).

Revisiting the orthodox categories view; benefits and evidence-based responses to challenges

Orthodox position on categories

An orthodox view is that schizophrenia is usefully and justifiably recognised as a category of mental disorder. Furthermore, in a wide category such as 'mental disorder,' distinctions can be made between wellness and disorder. Within the broad group of mental disorders, one can identify categories such as 'psychotic disorders,' or 'depression.' Also, within groupings like 'psychotic disorders' there are distinctions between different types for example, 'brief psychotic disorder' and 'schizophrenia.' This position is reflected in the guidance of *DSM-5* (American Psychiatric Association, 2013, passim) and of *ICD-11* (World Health Organisation, 2021, passim).

Benefits of classification

A strong case remains for retaining the term, concept and definition of schizophrenia while recognising its complex relationships to other conditions. As Torrey (2019, p. 55) emphasises, it is important to develop strong definitions so that suitable treatment can be provided, an individual with schizophrenia and their family can be given a prognosis, and different researchers can have confidence that they are studying the same disorder (Torrey, 2019, p. 55). More broadly, classification also allows better communication among professionals and between professionals, patients, and their families.

Evidence-based responses to challenges of categorisation

An orthodox position does not ignore relevant criticisms such as that schizophrenia is 'defined operationally, is encroached by neighbouring entities, and still lacks identity validation' (Stefanis and Stefanis, 2009, p. 1). Research aims to improve the usefulness of the category of schizophrenia, including the validity and reliability of classification and of diagnoses.

Refinements continue to accrue. Recall that, in *DSM-5* (American Psychiatric Association, 2013, p. 99) schizophrenia is distinguished from other psychotic disorders in several ways relating to the breadth of its symptoms, and its scope, severity, and duration. As well, there is a comparatively recent diagnostic requirement that two or more of the key symptoms of hallucinations, delusions, or disordered speech are evident.

Furthermore, 'paranoid schizophrenia,' once classified as a subtype of schizophrenia, was problematic. It was found to have limited stability as diagnoses, low reliability, and poor validity, and was unhelpful in diagnosis or treatment. As a result, in 2013, *DSM-5* reenvisaged paranoia (delusions of persecution) as a symptom of schizophrenia rather than a sub-type.

When evidence indicates problems, this is recognised, as with schizoaffective disorder for which *DSM-5* notes growing evidence that it is not 'a distinctive nosological category' (American Psychiatric Association, 2013, p. 90). There are already conditions that reflect the role of mood in psychosis. It is recognised that differential diagnosis of schizophrenia and bipolar disorders involves careful distinctions. Schizophrenia-related changes in mood can involve mania and depression, but these typically do not meet the criteria for full-blown mania or depression as in bipolar disorder (Altamura et al., 2009, p. 52).

In brief, the concept of schizophrenia continues to be useful and is gradually being refined in the light of new evidence. This approach makes some of the more voluble criticisms of it as a concept seem overstated and misguided.

Conclusion

Key internationally used psychiatric guidance reflects the orthodox position that schizophrenia is a category of disorder. Difficulties arise in securely establishing validity and reliability of schizophrenia. There are challenges of schizophrenia being defined operationally and being encroached by related conditions; and schizophrenia having no single cause and the different causes not always being present. Also, psychotic disorders defined by symptoms are potentially misleading because different disorders can produce the same symptoms, while no single symptom securely identifies schizophrenia. Furthermore, although schizophrenia is seen as categorical, psychotic illness appears more permeating, discouraging a too rigid separation between mental disorders. Orthodox practitioners take the view that these challenges can be met, while dissenters consider then insurmountable.

Turning to other criticisms, dissenters claim that schizophrenia was invented by pioneers Kraepelin and Bleuler but supporting argument is weak, drawing on emotive language and euphemism. Another criticism is that the conceptualisation of schizophrenia lacks scientific rigour. This presents an orthodox categorical view as based on false assumptions that madness can be divided into a few diseases, and that symptoms of madness cannot be understood in terms of the person's psychology. Maintaining that these are not assumptions but propositions that can be examined and tested, I suggest that the criticism is overstated and unfounded.

Dissenters have put forward alternatives to categorisation. One is proposing a continuum between wellness and schizophrenia having no firm dividing lines. However, symptoms of psychosis are generally very different to what most people experience day to day. Another alternative is a symptoms-based approach. This focuses on identifiable groups of symptoms 'within' schizophrenia that tend to occur together, like hallucinations. While it may be used for assessment and treatment, its reliability is questioned.

The chapter endorses the orthodox position of retaining the concept of schizophrenia. This involves recognising where criticism is justifiable, and responding accordingly and refining the concept of schizophrenia according to new evidence.

Suggested further reading

American Psychiatric Association (2013) *Diagnostic and Statistical Manual of Mental Disorders Fifth Edition (DSM-5)*. Washington DC, APA.

Kwapil, T. R. and Barrantes-Vidal, N. (2015) 'Schizotypy: Looking back and moving forward' *Schizophrenia Bulletin* 41, 2, S366–S373.

References

Altamura, C. A., Dragogna, F., Pozzoli, S. and Mauri, M. C. (2009) 'Schizophrenia: Differential diagnosis and comorbidities' in Kasper, S. and Papadimitriou, G. N. (Eds.) (2nd Edition) *Schizophrenia: Biopsychosocial Approaches and Current Challenges* (Medical Psychiatry Series). New York and London, Informa Healthcare (pp. 52–69).

American Psychiatric Association (2013) *Diagnostic and Statistical Manual of Mental Disorders Fifth Edition (DSM5)*. Washington DC, APA.

Bentall, R. (2003) *Madness Explained: Psychosis and Human Nature*. London, Penguin Books.

Carter, D. M., McKinnon, A., Howard, S., Zeegers, T. and Copolov, D. L. (1995) 'The development and reliability of the Mental Health Research Institute Unusual Perceptions Schedule MUPS): An instrument to record auditory hallucinatory experiences' *Schizophrenia Research* 16, 157–165.

Cohen, A. S. and Docherty, N. M. (2005) 'Symptom orientated versus syndrome approaches to resolving heterogeneity of neuropsychological functioning in schizophrenia' *Neuropsychiatry* 17, 3, 384–390. https://neuro.psychiatryonline.org/doi/10.1176/jnp.17.3.384

Cooke, A. (Ed.) (2017) *Understanding Psychosis and Schizophrenia: Why people sometimes hear voices, believe things that others find strange, or appear out of touch with reality, and what can help*. British Psychological Society Division of Clinical Psychology/Canterbury Christchurch University.

Hogan, M. (2010) 'Updated schizophrenia PORT treatment recommendations: A commentary' *Schizophrenia Bulletin* 36, 1, 104–106. https://www.ncbi.nlm.nih.gov/pmc/articles/PMC2800148/pdf/sbp127.pdf

Kirkpatrick, B., Buchanan, R. W., Ross, D. E. and Carpenter, W. T. (2001) 'A separate disease within the syndrome of schizophrenia' *Archives of General Psychiatry* 58, 2, 165–171.

Kreyenbuhl, J., Buchanan, R. W., Dickerson, F. B. and Dixon, L. B. (2010) 'The Schizophrenia Patient Outcomes Research Team (PORT): Updated treatment recommendations 2009' *Schizophrenia Bulletin* 36, 1, 94–103 January. https://www.ncbi.nlm.nih.gov/pmc/articles/PMC2800150/

Kwapil, T. R. and Barrantes-Vidal, N. (2015) 'Schizotypy: Looking back and moving forward' *Schizophrenia Bulletin* 41, 2, S366–S373.

Mojtabai, R. and Rieder, R. O. (1998) 'Limitations of the symptom-orientated approach to psychiatric research' *British Journal of Psychiatry* 173, 198–202.

Murray, R. and Dean, K. (2008) (4th Edition) 'Schizophrenia and related disorders' in Murray, R., Kendler, K., McGuffin, P., Wesseley, S. and Castle, D. (Eds.) *Essential Psychiatry*. Cambridge, Cambridge University Press.

National Institute of Mental Health (accessed January 2022) Schizophrenia May 2020 revision. https://www.nimh.nih.gov/health/topics/schizophrenia

NICE (2014) *Psychosis and schizophrenia in adults: prevention and management.* Clinical guidelines 12 February 2014. www.nice.org.uk/guidance/cg178

Read, J. (2013a) 'The invention of "schizophrenia": Kraepelin and Bleuler' in Read, J. and Dillon, J. (Eds.) (2nd Edition) *Models of Madness: Psychological, Social and Biological Approaches to Psychosis*. London and New York, Routledge (pp. 20–33).

Rutter, M., Nemeroff, C. B., Weinberger, D., Rutter, M., MacMillan, H. L., Bryant, R. A., Wessely, S., Stein, D. J., Pariante, C. M., Seemüller, F., Berk, M., Malhi, G. S., Preisig, M., Brüne, M. and Lysaker, P. (2013) 'DSM-5: A collection of psychiatrist views on the changes, controversies, and future directions' *School of Medicine, Johns Hopkins University* 13 September 2013. https://jhu.pure.elsevier.com/en/organisations/school-of-medicine-3

Skull, A. (2011) *Madness: A Very Short Introduction*. Oxford, Oxford University Press.

Stefanis, C. N. and Stefanis, N. C. (2009) 'Schizophrenia: Historical roots and brief review of recent research developments' in Kasper, S. and Papadimitriou, G. N. (Eds.) (2nd Edition) *Schizophrenia: Biopsychosocial Approaches and Current Challenges* (Medical Psychiatry Series). New York and London, Informa Healthcare (pp. 1–16).

Strauss, G. P., Harrow, M., Grossman, L. S. and Rosen, C. (2010) 'Periods of recovery in deficit syndrome schizophrenia' *Schizophrenia Bulletin* 36, 788–799.

Torrey, E. F. (2019) (7th Edition) *Surviving Schizophrenia: A Family Manual*. New York and London, Harper Perennial.

Valle, R. (2020) 'Schizophrenia in ICD-11: Comparison of ICD-10 and DSM-5' *Journal of Psychiatry and Mental Health* 13, 2, 95–104 April-June 2020 (translated from the Spanish). https://www.elsevier.es/en-revista-revista-psiquiatria-salud-mental-486-articulo-schizophrenia-in-icd-11-comparison-icd-10-S2173505020300145

World Health Organisation (2021) *International Statistical Classification of Diseases and Related Health Problems – eleventh iteration (ICD-11)*. World Health Organisation. https://www.who.int/standards/classifications/classification-of-diseases

3

A BIOPSYCHOSOCIAL PERSPECTIVE OF SCHIZOPHRENIA

Introduction

An orthodox biopsychosocial understanding of schizophrenia identifies it as a brain disorder understood, approached, and described in medical terms. At the same time, psychological and social factors are taken into account in understanding causation, and in treatment.

Critics of an orthodox approach to schizophrenia may emphasise the physical aspects of a biopsychosocial perspective, conveyed by the term, 'medical model' used with negative connotations. Accordingly, they may claim that regarding schizophrenia as a physical illness, assumes that it therefore requires solely physical treatment like medication, or electro-convulsive therapy (ECT). However, an orthodox position recognises not only physical causal factors, but also environmental and social triggers that can precipitate schizophrenia. Furthermore, it recognises the place of nonphysical treatments.

Another criticism is that a medical approach is pessimistic about the chances of recovery from schizophrenia. The condition is depicted as an incurable illness, and a life-long brain disease in which life events and circumstances can play no causal role. However, evidence of the long-term progress of people with schizophrenia does not support this position.

Critics may take a subjectivist view in which knowledge is personal and there is no external or objective truth. Accordingly, positions are not examined for evidence of whether they are true or correct. On the contrary, they are presented as what 'some people' think or feel and what 'others' think or feel as though personal and subjective views and experiences imply

DOI: 10.4324/9781003413554-3

objective, agreed truth. Relatedly, understanding schizophrenia as an illness is regarded as just another theory. Criticism is sometimes expressed in rhetoric such as an emphasis on the simplistic, outdated, reductionist, unsubstantiated, contextless, and crude, and a resort to emotive language.

Orthodox and dissenting positions

An orthodox position sees schizophrenia in medical terms. It is, 'a serious mental illness' affecting thinking, feelings, and behaviour (National Institute of Mental Health, accessed January 2022). It is, 'a disease of the brain' and 'a real (physical) disease' like other physical conditions such as high blood pressure (Kasper and Papadimitriou, 2009, p. xiii). Medical terminology tends to be used such as schizophrenia being 'diagnosed,' having 'symptoms,' and the chances of 'recovery' (Torrey, 2019, p. 85). At the same time, there is clear acceptance that psychological and social factors contribute to causes of schizophrenia. Also, treatment involves, 'the use of psychosocial interventions' as well as drugs. This reflects current recommendations from 'academic, clinical, and institutional settings' (Granholm and Loh, 2009, p. 270).

In a dissenting position, schizophrenia is not seen medically. Indications like 'unusual experiences' that are 'currently labelled' as schizophrenia are not regarded as 'symptoms of a medical illness.' Dissenters speak disapprovingly of a 'medical model' of schizophrenia which they consider to be too dominant (Read, Mosher and Bentall, 2013, p. 3). Similarly, it is said that experiences like hearing voices can lead to distress, but this does not mean that they are 'necessarily symptoms of real "illnesses."' (Cooke, 2017, section 3.4.1). Taking a relativist perspective calling such experiences schizophrenia, is seen as just 'one way of thinking about them' (Ibid., p. 6, executive summary).

A biopsychosocial approach to schizophrenia

As editors of a medical psychiatric textbook, Kasper and Papadimitriou (2009, p. xiii) state, 'Schizophrenia is a disease of the brain.' Also, it is worth highlighting that it is 'a real (physical) disease like diabetes, epilepsy, or high blood pressure' (Ibid., p. xiii). Along similar lines, Torrey (2019, p. 59) notes that there are many 'abnormalities in brain structure and function' that can be associated with schizophrenia, but no single, measurable feature that can confirm the condition. It is also likely that schizophrenia encompasses more than one 'disease entity' (Ibid.).

As a medical condition, schizophrenia is seen in terms of diagnosis, aetiology, treatment, prognosis, and recovery. Certainly, a causal view of schizophrenia as a disease or illness is concerned with physical, biological, and neurological factors including genetic aspects, and brain morphology and functioning. At the same time, psychological, family, and wider social factors are recognised. In the treatment of schizophrenia, physical interventions such as medication are important, but so are psychological and social approaches like family support.

Clinicians and researchers identify positive predictive aspects to a medical view. As Torrey (2019) points out, when someone is initially diagnosed with schizophrenia, they and their family are likely to have many questions. These may include wanting to know the chances of the individual making a full recovery and asking questions about the future such as, 'How independent is the person likely to be ten years later, or thirty years later?' (Ibid., p. 85).

Identification and diagnosis are complex but provide access to knowledge of how schizophrenia has affected others, what might be expected, and the possibilities for treatment and support. At a practical level, a diagnosis of schizophrenia can give access to health insurance and other financial help. It can also put families who have a member with schizophrenia in touch with other families in the same position so that mutual support can be offered.

As we will see below, critics of a biopsychosocial view of schizophrenia may play down psychosocial elements and emphasise physical aspects. Having distorted the perspective, they may call it a 'medical model' perhaps adding terms like 'simplistic.'

Criticisms that physical causes demand physical treatments – illogical, and unsupported by evidence

Criticisms that physical causes demand physical treatment for schizophrenia

Critics may claim that those regarding schizophrenia as a physical illness, assume that it therefore requires solely physical treatment like medication, or ECT. They refer to a 'misguided but powerful minority.' This group announces, drawing on the accoutrements of scientific and professional authority, that schizophrenia is an illness, so people with the disorder are told that they 'must take the drugs, by force, if necessary' (Read, Mosher and Bentall, 2013, p. 5). Also, genetic theories are presented as 'simplistic and reductionist.' They have been acted upon in spite of the accompanying high risks and the limited good quality research demonstrating effectiveness. This has led to 'the lobotomising, electroshocking or drugging of millions of people' (Ibid., p. 3). Too often, it is claimed, 'the only solution offered is a chemical or electrical one, usually delivered in a dehumanising prison-like hospital' (Ibid., p. 4).

Relatedly, Cooke (2017) suggests that when difficult decisions must be made there is a temptation to depend upon, 'a simplistic medical model.' It may be assumed that 'this person has no insight into their illness, so they need to be detained and administered medication, by force if necessary' (Ibid., p. 103, section 13.1). Campbell (2010) speaks of his gradual dis-illusionment with a 'medical model' which emphasised distress and en-couraged turning to, 'exclusively physical treatments' (Ibid.).

David Oaks on the MindFreedom International website (https://mindfreedom.org/kb/not-mentally-ill/) rejects the term 'mentally ill' maintaining that it reflects a constrained medical model. Where used about others including 'psychiatric survivors' it can be unwelcome, implying that, 'since "illness" is the problem, then a physician ought to be part of the solution.' Also, if mental illness is like a 'materialistic physical illness' this might imply that 'the solution ought to be physical too, such as a chemical or a drug or electricity.'

However, the claim that clinicians are locked into an approach that sees schizophrenia as a physical disease which therefore commits them to a physical treatment is illogical and unsupported by evidence.

Physical causes are only part of the picture

Information provided by the National Health Service in England (NHS, reviewed by them in 2019) touches on possible physical causal factors. Genes are recognised to be, 'not the only factor influencing the development of schizophrenia.' Studies of brain development and structure suggest that 'schizophrenia may partly be a disorder of the brain.' It is recognised that there is 'a connection between neurotransmitters and schizophrenia' for example because drugs altering the levels of brain neurotransmitters relieve some schizophrenia symptoms.

At the same time, other causal factors are highlighted. For instance, research shows that people developing schizophrenia are more likely to have experienced complications before and during their birth, like low birthweight, premature labour, and asphyxia during birth. These factors may exert a subtle effect on brain development (NHS, reviewed 2019).

In individuals who are at risk, certain triggers can precipitate schizo-phrenia. Such psychological triggers include stressful life events like bereavement, loss of job or home, divorce, the end of a relationship, and physical, sexual, or emotional abuse. Drugs do not directly cause schizo-phrenia, but their misuse increases the risk of developing the disorder. For example, drugs such as cannabis, lysergic acid diethylamide (LSD), or amphetamines can trigger symptoms of schizophrenia in susceptible people (NHS, reviewed by them in 2019).

In brief, although the 'exact' causes of schizophrenia are unknown, research indicates that 'a combination of physical, genetic, psychological and environmental factors' can increase the risk of someone developing the disorder. Proneness to schizophrenia is mentioned noting that, 'a stressful or emotional life event might trigger a psychotic episode' (NHS, reviewed 2019).

Nonphysical treatments form part of the repertoire of an orthodox approach

Acknowledgements of the importance of physical, psychological, social, and environmental factors is reflected in the term 'biopsychosocial' perspective. Some critics are still unconvinced by the development of such an approach. For them, the expression 'biopsychosocial' has only given the illusion of an integration of models because the 'vulnerability-stress' idea within this approach relegates life-events, '... to the role of "triggers" of an underlying genetic timebomb' (Read and Dillon, 2013, p. 4).

These critics take the view that this perceived relegation of life events represents a 'colonisation of the psychological and social by the biological' which has involved '... the ignoring, or vilification' of research implicating contextual factors. These factors may include stress, trauma, poverty, sexism, and racism in seeking to explain how psychosis emerges (Read and Dillon, 2013, p. 4). Yet there are many examples of orthodox practitioners recognising the importance of psychological and social influences in schizophrenia. This cannot justifiably be represented as ignoring contextual factors or their vilification.

Torrey (2019, p. 198), taking a medical perspective of schizophrenia, discusses several alternatives to drugs or ECT. Regarding herbal treatments, he refers to a social survey that had found that 22% of people with 'mania or psychosis' had taken some kind of alternative medicine including herbal remedies in the past 12 months (Unützer et al., 2000). Torrey (2019) mentions for example ginkgo biloba (a leaf extract used as a dietary supplement) used to treat 'cognitive symptoms' of schizophrenia. He does however advise that people with schizophrenia should exercise caution towards herbal treatments (Ibid., p. 198). Discussing cognitive-behavioural therapy he notes that it is 'popular for treating the positive symptoms ... of schizophrenia' and that randomised trials suggest that it is 'modestly effective' in enabling patients to deal with delusions and hallucinations (Ibid., p. 200). Family therapy is also seen as an 'important component' for treating schizophrenia (Ibid., p. 201).

In their edited book, Kasper and Papadimitriou (2009), who make a point of emphasising that schizophrenia is a disease of the brain and a physical disease, include a chapter by Granholm and Loh (2013). Discussing evidence-based psychosocial interventions for schizophrenia the chapter refers to current recommendations for treating schizophrenia from 'academic, clinical, and institutional settings.' All these recommendations 'advocate for the use of psychosocial interventions in addition to pharmacology' when treating schizophrenia (Ibid., p. 270). Evidence-based interventions for schizophrenia are effective for a wide range of difficulties including 'cognitive impairments, positive and negative symptoms, and social and occupational functioning' (Ibid.).

Granholm and Loh (2013, pp. 270–274) discuss a range of recommended provision. This includes *family interventions* that may be delivered family to family. In '*supported employment*' the person's interests and choice are important, and a special counsellor helps in finding competitive employment in an integrated setting with salaries at or above minimum national wage. Involving flexibility and multidisciplinary collaboration, Assertive Community Treatment ensures that all possible treatment is provided by an ACT team rather than in many centres.

Also considered is *social skills training* which aims to teach skills involved in elements of social competence to improve interpersonal communication and effectiveness. Cognitive-behavioural therapy as applied to schizophrenia can challenge beliefs about psychotic symptoms, social aversion attitudes, and defeatist performance beliefs that interfere with community functioning. Also discussed are various other 'promising' psychosocial interventions for schizophrenia (Granholm and Loh, 2013, pp. 274–276).

Criticism that the 'medical model' is pessimistic – overlooking contrary evidence

Dissenters castigate a medical model for seeming pessimism about the chances of recovery from schizophrenia, related to the condition being viewed as an incurable illness, and a life-long brain disease. Some claim that because schizophrenia is believed to be an illness 'therefore, life events and circumstances can play no role in its causation' (Read, Mosher and Bentall, 2013, p. 4). Fallaciously, the argument continues that this has led to 'the awful conclusion that nothing can be done to prevent it.' Consequently, biological psychiatry 'gives politicians a perfect excuse for doing nothing' (Ibid.).

Critics suggest that seeing schizophrenia as a disease diminishes the importance of other factors such as the family and social context. The medical model of schizophrenia, they state, has too long 'dominated efforts to understand and assist distressed and distressing people.' It is responsible for 'unwarranted and destructive pessimism' about the possibilities of recovery. The model has taken no account of the events in these people's lives, or their family and social context (Read, Mosher and Bentall, 2013, p. 3).

It is intimated that a medical approach can rob people of their feelings of control over their lives and can lead to individuals being negatively labelled. Campbell (2010) speaks of his gradual disillusionment with a medical model which encouraged a view of 'having a chronic and incurable illness,' took away his 'power of agency' and confined him 'within an essentially negative category' (Ibid., p. 22). Sally Edwards (quoted in Cooke, 2017) speaks approvingly of joining a self-help group whose members accepted her experiences as part of her identity rather than as 'part of a medical illness' Edwards adds, 'I didn't believe I was a psychiatric patient with a lifelong brain disease any more ...' (Ibid., section 9.2.1).

However, the idea of a life-long incurable brain disease creating a destructive pessimism about recovery is itself over pessimistic. A study reported the prognosis at the end of one year of 77 patients hospitalised with schizophrenia disorder (including schizoaffective disorder) for the first time (Lieberman et al., 1993). Some 74% were considered 'fully re-mitted' and 12% 'partially remitted.'

Looking at long-term follow-up and prognosis for schizophrenia, Stephens (1978) analysed, 25 studies in which there had been follow-up for ten years or more. The broad picture was that:

- 25% recover completely
- 25% are much improved (can live relatively independently, may marry, and can often work full or part-time)
- 25% are modestly improved (require an extensive support network, and where this is not available may struggle)
- 15% are unimproved, and
- 10% are dead mostly from suicide.

Notably, the studies varied considerably according to the percentage of patients 'recovered,' 'improved,' or 'unimproved.' This in turn depended on how patients were initially selected. For example, the higher the numbers with acute reactive psychosis, the greater the percentage fully recovered. The figure of 25% recovered completely, encompasses all pa-tients with symptoms of schizophrenia in the analysis. This includes those who had been affected for less than six months with schizophreniform disorders. If a tighter definition of schizophrenia is used, with continuous signs of disorder for at least six months, the percentage completely re-covered falls below 25% (see also Torrey, 2019, pp. 97–100). Regarding patients followed up for an average of 36 years, about three-fifths of those with schizophrenia recover or show definite improvement (Ciompi, 1980).

Harding and colleagues (Harding and Strauss, 1985; Harding et al., 1987) carried out a 32-year longitudinal study of 269 'back-ward' patients from Vermont State Hospital. This is old research, but inevitably tied to the past because it involved a historical period when institutions were being run down. The cohort took part in a wide-ranging rehabilitation programme. Patients were released into the community during the 1950s as part of the trend for deinstitutionalisation.

At ten years follow-up, 70% of these patients remained out of the hospital although many were socially isolated or were recidivists. Twenty to 25 years after their index release, a further assessment was carried out on 262 of these individuals. They were blindly assessed with structured, reliable protocols. A half to two-thirds of this group had achieved 'considerable improvement or recovery' (Harding et al., 1987). The authors note that this finding corroborated similar findings from Europe and elsewhere.

In reviewing these findings, Torrey (2019) put the view that a highly pessimistic representation of schizophrenia is a caricature. He argues that recent research has clearly established that, for the average patient, the 30-year course of schizophrenia is more favourable than the ten-year course. Such research, he concludes, 'directly contradicts a widespread stereotype of the disease that dates to Kraepelin's pessimistic belief that most patients slowly deteriorate' (Ibid., p. 101).

Proposing subjectivism over medical evidence – self-refuting and lacking significance

Subjectivism

A view that subjective personal views (subjectivism) are just as valid as medical ones is sometimes presented to criticise the latter. Subjectivism (sometimes referred to as subjective relativism) relates to the wider perspective of relativism. In brief, relativism is the claim that standards of truth, rationality, and right and wrong vary between cultures and historical periods. Accordingly, no 'universal criteria' exist for adjudicating between such standards. However, relativism is criticised for inconsistency, because if the statement 'truth is relative' is understood as an unconditional claim, it is self-refuting. If the statement is interpreted relativistically it is 'devoid of significance' (Baghramian, 2001, abstract).

Within this context, subjectivism is the view that knowledge is subjective and personal and that there is no external or objective truth. This is because different people have different beliefs and perceptions about knowledge (and morality). So, what is true (or right or wrong) for one person may not be true (or right or wrong) for another. A criticism of subjectivism, parallel to that of relativism, is that if 'truth is subjective' is taken as an unconditional claim it is self-refuting; if interpreted subjectively it has no significance.

An indication of subjectivism is found when positions are not examined for evidence of whether they are true or correct. Someone may narcissistically speak of 'my truth' as if it were comparable with demonstrable truth. In the context of discussions about schizophrenia and related matters, positions are presented as what 'some people' think or feel and what 'others' think or feel. This can suggest that personal and subjective views and experiences imply truth. Another implication is that, because there are different views of what constitutes truth, it is not possible to be definitive. All that commentators can do is observe that some people say this, and other people say that without any attempt to evaluate the respective claims.

Schizophrenia and psychosis and subjectivism

The report *Understanding Psychosis and Schizophrenia* (Cooke, 2017) provides exhaustive examples of subjectivism. A few may suffice. The document states that 'Some people find it useful to think of themselves as having an illness. Others prefer to think of their problems as, for example, an aspect of their personality' (Ibid., p. 6, executive summary). Traditionally, paranoia, or hearing voices not heard by others have been regarded as indications of mental illness. However, 'Some people find it helpful to think of their problems as an illness, but others do not' (Ibid., p. 7, note on terminology). Professionals should 'support people in whatever way they personally find most helpful ...' (Ibid., p. 103).

Where the report does take a position rather than just saying what 'some people' think or feel, or find helpful, it discourages any insistence that schizophrenia is an illness. Indeed, professionals 'should not insist that people agree with the view that experiences are symptoms of an underlying illness' (Ibid., p. 105).

What is important in the report is not so much whether schizophrenia (or psychosis) is an illness according to evidence such as that from genetics, brain morphology, and neurochemical findings. What is central is whether people 'think of themselves' as having an illness (Ibid., p. 6, executive summary); whether they 'find this a helpful way of understanding what is going on' (Ibid., p. 7, note on terminology); or whether they 'find it helpful to think of their problems as an illness' (Ibid., p. 103).

Proposing that seeing schizophrenia as an illness is just another theory – underplaying evidence

Related to these examples of subjectivism, the report *Understanding Psychosis and Schizophrenia* (Cooke, 2017) diminishes the importance of a medical approach. It does this by proposing that the perspective is merely one view among many, and that other views might carry equal or greater weight. It says that regarding hearing voices, referring to them in medical terms such as symptoms of schizophrenia is only 'one way of thinking about them' (Cooke, 2017, p. 6, Executive Summary). The report reflects that many different theories exist about the causes of experiences like hearing voices that others do not hear. Any notion that such experiences are illness symptoms, that may be brought about by 'chemical imbalance or other problem in the brain' is merely 'just one of the theories' (Ibid., p. 17, section 3, Introduction).

Yet surely such a claim underplays the role of evidence from observation or research that one view is more accurate (or more in line with the evidence) than another. Instead, one is invited to accept that everyone might have a different view and no one person's view is any better than another's. To simply say that 'some people' say this or that avoids judgement and evaluation about what is said.

Regarding psychosis, a key issue is the evidence that one view or the other is correct. A scientific approach is interested in such matters, while a subjectivist view can simply present the range of opinions. Explanations that psychosis relates to some 'problem in the brain,' so long as that problem is specified, can be tested, and found to be correct or incorrect. It is not 'just another theory' in that sense. Attempted explanations can be judged to be correct or accurate or at least plausible to different degrees. They are not solely based on just what 'some people' find a helpful way to think about things.

Emphasising the simplistic, outdated, reductionist, unsubstantiated, contextless, and crude – criticising the weakest scenario

Cooke (2017, section 13.1) criticises the temptation to rely on 'a simplistic medical model' which is supposed to imply that patients need 'to be detained and administered medication, by force if necessary' (Ibid.). Sally Edwards (quoted in Cooke, 2017, section 9.2.1) speaks of being 'an activist' who wants to change the present system which is founded on an 'outdated medical model' (Ibid.).

Read, Mosher and Bentall (2013, pp. 3–8) mention 'Simplistic and reductionist genetic and biological theories' leading to 'lobotomising, electroshocking or drugging of millions of people' (Ibid., p. 3). We should eschew '... unsubstantiated bio-genetic ideologies and technologies' (Ibid., p. 3). Furthermore, such critics say that some medical professionals are too ready to believe that the complicated nature of human experience can be grasped through a 'single, contextless, medical sounding word' (Ibid., p. 4). Such orthodox clinicians and researchers try to explain madness using the 'crude concepts and tools of biological psychiatry ...' (Ibid., p. 5).

But do mental health professionals (or anyone else) adhere to models and approaches that are simplistic, outdated, reductionist, unsubstantiated, contextless, and crude? If so, this is (by definition) not a good thing. But who today endorses a simplistic rather than a nuanced medical approach? Who among psychiatrists really believes that the complexities of human experience are captured in a single word, even if it is medical sounding? Which researchers boast cleaving to 'outdated' and 'unsubstantiated' claims rather than up to date evidence-based proposals?

As a rhetorical device, narrowing criticism to a model or approach that is self-evidently weak, blunts the point. It paints a flattering picture of dissenters as people who can distinguish the simplistic, outdated, reductionist, unsubstantiated, contextless, and crude and can presumably instead present the complex, contemporary, confirmed, contextual, and sophisticated. But such criticism might be more telling if it attempted to engage with current medical approaches that emphasise biological factors in schizophrenia but also take account of psychological and social influences.

Criticism using exaggerated and emotive language

Read, Mosher and Bentall (2013) in a book chapter titled 'Schizophrenia is not an illness' (Ibid., pp. 3–8) typify some of the exaggerated and emotive language that muddies debate. Metaphor and simile draw on incarceration, explosives, the notion of imperialism and occupying forces, and hatred. Hospitals are 'dehumanising prison-like' places (Ibid., p. 4). Life events become 'triggers of an underlying genetic timebomb' (Ibid.). The dominance of a biological view reflects '... a colonisation of the psychological and social by the biological' which has involved the 'vilification' of research which indicates how social and environmental context contribute to the origins of psychosis (Ibid.).

In such criticisms, important questions and debates may be alluded to but not in language that illuminates issues or carries the argument forward. How does the view of schizophrenia as an illness lead to the 'awful conclusion' that nothing can be done to prevent it? To whom exactly does 'biological psychiatry' refer and how do their views give politicians 'a perfect excuse for doing nothing' (Read, Mosher and Bentall, 2013, p. 4). How does the emotiveness of saying that 'Tens of thousands' are having 'electric shocks applied to their brains to cause convulsions in the name of "psychiatric treatment"' (Ibid., p. 5) engage with debates about the effectiveness or otherwise of the contemporary use of ECT? Exaggerated and emotive language is unconvincing and lacking in argument.

Conclusion

A medical approach identifies schizophrenia as an illness emphasising biological and physical factors, but recognising psychological, family, and wider social elements. Seeing schizophrenia as a medical condition implies a context of diagnosis, aetiology, course, treatment, prognosis, and related understanding and terminology. For those trying to understand and respond to schizophrenia, this context can provide a framework based on a physical and biological foundation, while recognising psychological and social factors. A medical diagnosis can give the person diagnosed and their relatives and friends an indication of what to expect and can facilitate contact with help including support groups.

Critics may take a subjectivist view in which knowledge is subjective and personal and there is no external or objective truth. They examine positions not for evidence of whether they are true or correct but according to what 'some people' think or feel as though personal and subjective views and experiences imply truth. Relatedly, understanding schizophrenia as an illness is regarded as merely another theory.

Critics of a medical model see in it an unjustified pessimism about the outlook for people with schizophrenia and the outcome of the condition. While such a pessimism was a feature of historical perspectives, it unsupportable in the light of more recent research and developments which depict a more optimistic outlook for schizophrenia including in the long view.

Where schizophrenia is seen in biological and physical terms, it is sometimes said that this inevitably leads to the use of physical treatments such as medication. However, schizophrenia is not understood in exclusively physical terms, but account is taken of environmental and other factors. Also, treatment of schizophrenia is not restricted to physical ones like medication, although this is the most common intervention.

Rhetoric sometimes used in criticisms of a medical approach includes presenting medical perspectives as solely crude and simplistic which weakens the criticism for two reasons. Firstly, by definition, anyone would reject something that is too crude or simplistic such as believing that the complexity of human nature is distilled into a single medical sounding word. Secondly, where it is apparent that a medical view is not crude and simplistic but more nuanced, the criticism does not carry weight.

Where the language of criticism is exaggerated by the excessive use of negative adjectives, inflammatory metaphor and simile evoking prison, colonisation, and bombs, it clouds the issues. Where there is no precise target for criticism such as a psychiatrist or researcher who can put an alternative view and where instead the target is a nebulous one like 'biological psychiatry' the criticism is further weakened.

Suggested further reading

Cooke, A. (Ed.) (2017) *Understanding Psychosis and Schizophrenia: Why people sometimes hear voices, believe things that others find strange, or appear out of touch with reality, and what can help.* British Psychological Society Division of Clinical Psychology/Canterbury Christchurch University.

Torrey, E. F. (2019) (7th Edition) *Surviving Schizophrenia: A Family Manual.* New York and London, Harper Perennial.

References

Baghramian, M. (2011) 'Relativism: Philosophical aspects (Elsevier)' in Moser, P. K. and Carson, T. L. (Eds.) *The International Encyclopaedia of Behavioural and Social Sciences.* Elsevier.

Campbell, P. (2010) 'Surviving the system' in Basset, T. and Stickley, T. (Eds.) *Voices of Experience: Narratives of Mental Health Survivors.* Chichester, Wiley-Blackwell.

Ciompi, L. (1980) 'Catamnestic long-term study of the course of life and aging of schizophrenics' *Schizophrenia Bulletin* 6, 606–616. https://pubmed.ncbi.nlm.nih.gov/7444392/

Cooke, A. (Ed.) (2017) *Understanding Psychosis and Schizophrenia: Why people sometimes hear voices, believe things that others find strange, or appear out of touch with reality, and what can help.* British Psychological Society Division of Clinical Psychology/Canterbury Christchurch University.

Granholm, E. and Loh, K. (2009) 'Evidence-based psychosocial interventions for schizophrenia' in Kasper, S. and Papadimitriou, G. N. (Eds.) (2nd Edition) *Schizophrenia: Biopsychosocial Approaches and Current Challenges* (Medical Psychiatry Series). New York and London, Informa Healthcare (pp. 269–281).

Harding, C. M., Brooks, G. W., Ashikaga, T., Strauss, J. S. and Breier, A. (1987) 'The Vermont longitudinal study of persons with severe mental illness, I: Methodology, study sample, and overall status 32 years later' *American Journal of Psychiatry* 144, 6, 718–725. https://pubmed.ncbi.nlm.nih.gov/3591991/

Harding, C. M. and Strauss, J. S. (1985) 'The course of schizophrenia: An evolving concept' in Alpert, M. (Ed.) *Controversies in Schizophrenia.* New York, Guilford Press.

Kasper, S. and Papadimitriou, G. N. (Eds.) (2009) (2nd Edition) *Schizophrenia: Biopsychosocial Approaches and Current Challenges* (Medical Psychiatry Series). New York and London, Informa Healthcare.

Lieberman, J., Jody, D., Geisler, S., Alvir, J., Loebel, A., Szymanski, S., Woerner, M. and Borenstein, M. (1993) 'Time course and biologic correlates of treatment response in first-episode schizophrenia' *Archives of General Psychiatry* 50, 369–376. https://pubmed.ncbi.nlm.nih.gov/8098203/

National Institute of Mental Health (accessed 2022) *Assertive Community Treatment.* https://www.nimh.nih.gov/

NHS (reviewed November, 2019) *Schizophrenia Causes.* https://www.nhs.uk/mental-health/conditions/schizophrenia/causes/

Read, J. and Dillon, J. (Eds.) (2013) (2nd Edition) *Models of Madness: Psychological, Social and Biological Approaches to Psychosis*. London and New York, Routledge.

Read, J., Mosher, L. and Bentall, R. (2013) 'Schizophrenia is not an illness' in Read, J. and Dillon, J. (Eds.) (2013) (2nd Edition) *Models of Madness: Psychological, Social and Biological Approaches to Psychosis*. London and New York, Routledge (pp. 3–8).

Stephens, J. H. (1978) 'Long-term prognosis and follow-up in schizophrenia' *Schizophrenia Bulletin* 4, 25–47. https://psycnet.apa.org/record/2005-09716-009

Torrey, E. F. (2019) (7th Edition) *Surviving Schizophrenia: A Family Manual*. New York and London, Harper Perennial.

Unützer, J., Klap, R., Sturm, R., Young, A. S., Marmon, T., Shatkin, J. and Wells, K. B. (2000) 'Mental disorders and the use of alternative medicine: Results from a national survey' *American Journal of Psychiatry* 157, 1851–1857. https://pubmed.ncbi.nlm.nih.gov/11058485/

4

STIGMA AND SCHIZOPHRENIA

Introduction

Firstly, this chapter considers stigma and its mainly unfavourable associations including negative labelling and perceptions. I then examine the orthodox view that stigma is associated with the incidence of comparatively rare violence perpetrated by people with schizophrenia.. This includes evidence that individuals with schizophrenia are at an increased risk for perpetrating harm when compared with other people.

Focusing on criminal records, the chapter argues, can underestimate the prevalence of aggressive behaviour in schizophrenia, and the burden on family and professionals of caring for those affected, and coping with the condition. I consider the negative impact of high-profile acts of violence on public perceptions of schizophrenia. While the chapter recognises the rarity of this, it also notes the impact on families and friends of victims killed by individuals with schizophrenia.

A criticism from a dissenting view attributes stigma towards schizophrenia to orthodox psychiatry. Accordingly, critics depict biopsychosocial psychiatry as 'biological psychiatry,' misrepresenting it as exclusively concerned with physical issues. In this context, I look at critics' mistrust of the marketing and research (and research funding) of certain drug companies. A further criticism is that biogenetic causal beliefs are associated with negative attitudes to schizophrenia, and psychosocial beliefs with positive attitudes. This view, I suggest, relates to weak research evidence and a polarised presentation of biological and social choices in studies.

DOI: 10.4324/9781003413554-4

Orthodox and dissenting positions

An orthodox view recognises a that violence is more commonly perpetrated by people with schizophrenia than it is by people without mental disorders. It is 'roughly twice as frequent when controlling for the substantial effects of comorbid substance abuse.' Among robust variables associated with such increased risk of violence are 'younger age, previous violence, antisocial traits, and medication non-adherence' (Appelbaum, 2019). When a person with psychosis does engage in such harm, their informal carers are more likely to be the targets, and the violence 'will often occur within the family home' (Onwumere, Zhou and Kuipers, 2018). Research in the United States and Europe indicate that the biggest single cause of stigma against people with mental disorder is 'episodes of violence.' Studies also suggest that it would be difficult to decrease stigma until such episodes decrease (Torrey, 2019, p. 398). Stigma is driven it is believed by 'high-profile violent attacks committed by a small number of people with schizophrenia.' Furthermore, nearly all of these people were not being treated at the time of the attacks (Ibid., p. 362).

In a dissenting position, it is believed that stigma emerges from the label of schizophrenia, and its negative associations. Health professionals, patients, and families have called for a change of name viewing the term schizophrenia as 'highly stigmatising and ... associated with hopelessness, violence and discrimination' (Valle, 2020, 'Discussion'). A stereotype of schizophrenia combines 'dangerousness and unpredictability' and a caricature of the violent madman remains. In fact, people with psychosis are more likely to be assaulted than to assault others (Read, Haslam and Magliano, 2013, p. 157). Mental disorders are seen as less responsive to treatment and more persistent and serious when 'framed as biological diseases.' This may suggest that depicting schizophrenia as an illness from which people never recover contributes to stigma. Seeing mental disorder as involving psychological and social stressors can lead to a 'healthier public perception' (Canadian Health Services Research Foundation, 2012, p. 3). Ironically, psychiatric campaigns aiming to reduce stigma towards mental disorders by depicting them as 'like any other biological disease' may have helped to increase stigma (Davies, 2013, p. 223).

Stigma, labelling and perception

Stigma and labelling

In a report on psychosis and schizophrenia, an anonymous contributor says, 'The name doesn't help. It's psycho.' To the contributor this meant, 'someone that goes killing people and ... does crazy things' (Cooke, 2017,

p. 33). While some regard labelling as entirely negative, others find the act of naming a mental disorder to have benefits. Referring to bipolar disorder, Falk (2010) asserts, 'I think I prefer my illness having a name because it makes me feel less lonely.' She also knows that there are others that are going through her 'misery' and that they live through the illness and 'make a meaningful existence with it' (Ibid., p. 32).

On learning the name of her 'distress,' Pembroke (2012) says that she felt a 'relief response.' But she admits that the label on its own does not relieve the pain. Neither does a label help the clinician or the person with the disorder to understand what is happening or what might help. For Pembroke, 'the labelled people are seen as inferior or less competent' and 'People become dependent and helpless with the treatments and labels' (Ibid., p. 36).

Such responses suggest that although the use of categories of mental disorder and related labels can be negative, but this is not always so. Nevertheless, it is worth recalling that categories refer to disorders rather than to individuals. Saying that a person has 'schizophrenia' does not inevitably have to categorise the individual solely in these terms. There will be many further ways in which the individual will be seen in relation to other possible groupings such as gender, ethnic group, age, interests, as well as individual characteristics.

Stigma and perceptions of mental phenomena

Related to labelling is the way that mental phenomena are perceived. Davies (2013) makes the point about relative judgements of mental phenomena regarding hearing voices. In a society where hearing voices is mainly associated with mental disorders, people who hear them must contend with the 'difficult idea' that they are 'psychologically unwell.' This might create 'additional anxiety' and a 'sense of abnormality.' Individuals must deal with how these phenomena are seen socially and how they are defined and managed (Ibid., p. 219).

However, in a society in which these experiences do not attract suspicion and may be seen as signs of 'divine inspiration' the response is likely to be much more positive. The individual will certainly have a 'less tortured relationship with their internal voices' making them 'freer from the burdens of shame and angst.' Davies observes that how people are 'marked' can influence feelings. Therefore, when one is trying to understand any human experience trying to make sense of any human experience it must always be related to 'the dominant myth,' defining and evaluating the experience (Ibid., p. 219).

For Davies (2013), this implies that if people change the 'myth' through which these states are comprehended, this can have therapeutic effects. It can be as beneficial as, 'taking a pill or undergoing therapy' (Ibid., p. 221). Also, many patients are said to report that, once they reject the 'psychiatric view,' they frequently no longer experience, the stigma that goes along with being identified as 'psychiatrically unwell' (Ibid., p. 221).

A difficulty with this view is that it underplays situations in which a person hears voices which are harmful. Voices may command people to harm themselves or others. They may constantly tell the individual that they are evil or worthless, increasing the risk of self-harm or suicide. Rejecting a 'psychiatric view' as Davies suggests, seems to be vacuous in such instances.

Violence perpetrated by people with schizophrenia

Rarity of violence perpetrated by people with schizophrenia and concerns it is exaggerated

In a Swedish population-based cohort, it was found that individuals with schizophrenia were nearly twice as likely to be victims of homicide as they were to be perpetrators (Crump et al., 2013). Also, instances of homicide and of manifesting violence generally are rare among individuals with mental disorders, the great majority of whom harm no one. A global study mentions criminal homicide among people with psychosis in only an indirect footnote presumably because of its rarity (United Nations Office on Drugs and Crime, 2013).

Some cases involve people with schizophrenia commit dramatic violence or random attacks, or both. Here, concern arises that reporting this may provoke prejudice towards individuals with mental disorders. Even unvarnished, factual accounts can be seen as potentially inflammatory and sensationalising. Those expressing such concerns may reiterate that people with mental disorder are more likely to be vulnerable to harm than to perpetrate it.

Higher than average (but still low) risk of people with schizophrenia perpetrating violence

Referring to violence perpetrated by people with schizophrenia, Rabun and Boyer (2009) state that the literature demonstrates that people with schizophrenia have 'an increased risk for violence compared to the general public' (Ibid., p. 333).

Whiting et al. (2021) carried out a review and meta-analysis of 24 studies from 15 countries. Associations were examined between schizophrenia spectrum disorders and violence manifested by adults and adolescents. Comparing people with schizophrenia spectrum disorders and the general population, the researchers sought to identify the absolute risk and the relative risk of being violent towards others.

Searching databases in any language from 1970 to 2021, the researchers included certain case-control and cohort studies. Risks were identified of individuals with schizophrenia spectrum disorders perpetrating 'interpersonal violence' and/or 'violent criminality.' This was compared with risks from a group of the general population who did not have these disorders. Violence towards others was established from official records, self-report and/or collateral report, or medical file review. It included 'any physical assault, robbery, sexual offences, illegal threats and intimidation, and arson' (Whiting et al., 2021).

Covering a period of four decades, the meta-analysis included 24 studies of perpetration of violence outcomes in 15 countries. Included were over 50,000 people with schizophrenia spectrum disorders with a mean age of 21 to 54 years at follow-up. Not all studies reported outcomes separately by sex, but of those that did, 19,976 were male and 14,275 were female. Risk of perpetrating harm, the meta-analysis indicated, was increased in people with schizophrenia spectrum disorders compared with community control individuals. New population based-longitudinal studies and sibling comparison designs confirm this finding (Whiting et al., 2021).

Drawing on a subgroup of register-based studies, researchers calculated the absolute risk of being violent for people with schizophrenia spectrum disorders. It was less than 1 in 20 in women and less than 1 in 4 in men over a 35-year period. In summary, people with schizophrenia and related disorders are at higher-than-average risk of committing violence but the overall risk is still 'modest.' Increasing the risk of being violent were other factors like drug/alcohol misuse, which could form a target for preventing such violence. This evidence also indicates the importance of healthcare provision in tackling substance misuse.

Schizophrenia and violence towards family members

One indication of violence carried out by people with schizophrenia (and done to them) is criminal records. However, as Wehring and Carpenter (2011) note that concentrating too much on criminal records greatly underestimates how much aggressive behaviour there is in relation to schizophrenia. Such a focus also underrates the 'burden' on those who care for the person showing aggression in coping with it which includes threats of violence, and violent acts. The impact of this falls on a range of others including 'family members, clinical care staff, those who share housing, police, and staffs of emergency rooms and jails' (Ibid.).

Reflecting this, a qualitative study explored the experiences of caregivers of aggressive patients with schizophrenia. Most caregivers experienced multiple types of aggression (verbal aggression, physical aggression, and damage to property). Similar findings were shown by some studies which revealed that aggression could take the form of verbal threats, threats with knives, punches, wrestling, and damage to property (Neha et al., 2021).

In Taiwan, Hsu and Tu (2014) conducted a qualitative study. They describe the experiences of aggression and violence among patients with schizophrenia towards their parents; and identify factors precipitating violence. Data was collected from in-depth interviews in 2011 with 14 hospitalised patients with schizophrenia. In the previous year, all had acted out aggression and violence towards their biological parents. Five themes were identified by the researchers:

- violence occurring beyond control in a particular situation translated into parent and patient's possible endangerment
- the repetitive nature of violence
- distress
- ineffective communication, and
- management of violence and help-seeking.

Repeated violence and tension, the authors noted, made both patient and parent feel 'uncontrollable.' They advised that health professionals should be more aware of the complexity of the phenomena and the interplay of factors that induced violence. Also suggested was comprehensive intervention to prevent it (Hsu and Tu, 2014).

Stigma towards schizophrenia relating to violence and the perceived risk of violence

Violence and schizophrenia

Posing the question, 'Why is stigma so strong despite better public understanding of mental illness?' a US report (US Department of Health and Human Service, 1999) gave its own answer, 'fear of violence.' The report states that those experiencing metal disorder, particularly people with psychosis, are regarded as being more violent than in the past. In short, 'the perception of people with psychosis as being dangerous is stronger today than in the past' (Ibid.).

Lack of education is not the force that is driving stigma claims (Torrey, 2019). It is rather, 'high-profile violent acts committed by a small number of people with schizophrenia' (Ibid., p. 362). In Germany there were a series of attacks on well-known officials by people with severe mental illness. Immediately following these public attacks was a 'marked increase in desired social distance from mentally ill people' which gradually decreased over the subsequent two years (Angermeyer and Matschinger, 1996).

A 2016 study compared news stories from two ten-year periods, 1995–2004 and 2005–2014 (McGinty et al., 2016). It examined the proportion of front page newspaper stories about interpersonal violence relating to severe mental illness. This coverage increased from 1% in the first period studied to 18% in the second period. That second decade included the reporting of two mass shootings, one by a person diagnosed with schizoaffective disorder (James Egan Holmes), the other involving an individual with schizophrenia (Jared Lee Loughner).

James Egan Holmes was responsible for the Aurora, Colorado, shooting, killing 12 people and injuring 70 others at a movie theatre on 20 July 2012. A psychiatrist testified that Holmes experienced schizoaffective disorder. Holmes's plea of not guilty by reason of insanity was accepted. In January 2011, Jared Lee Loughner carried out a mass shooting in Tucson killing six people, including a US district court judge and a nine-year-old girl. After his arrest, Loughner was diagnosed with 'paranoid schizophrenia' and ruled incompetent to stand trial. Judged competent to stand trial in August 2012, Loughner pleaded guilty to 19 counts.

Other examples of killings by people with mental disorder are widely published. In 2016, TASS reported that Gyulchehra Bobokulova was arrested in Moscow on suspicion of the 'atrocious murder of a four-year-old girl.' She told journalists in court that Allah ordered her to commit the brutal crime. According to investigators, on February 29 after the parents of the victim and their elder child left the apartment, the 38-year-old nanny 'for unknown reasons committed the murder, set the apartment on fire and escaped.' On the same day police officers detained the nanny by the Oktyabrskoye Pole subway station. She was walking about 'carrying the head of the killed child and threatening others with organizing an explosion' (TASS, 2016).

Alexander Lewis-Ranwell, 38, had been diagnosed with schizophrenia with delusions of persecution. On 10 February 2019, having left police custody in Barnstaple, England, he travelled to Exeter. There, he entered the private house of Anthony Paine, 80, and beat him to death with a hammer. Later entering the house of twins Dick Carter and Roger Carter, 84, he bludgeoned them to death with a spade. Lewis-Ranwell falsely believed that Anthony Paine was holding a kidnapped girl in his cellar, and that the Carter twins were implicated in child abuse and torture.

Found not guilty by reason of insanity Lewis-Ranwell was given a hospital restriction order (Dilley and Kemp, 2019; Morris, 2019).

The impact of violent acts relating to schizophrenia

Where some commentators discuss violence perpetrated by people with schizophrenia, they may provide a context for it. To those effected, this can be seen as minimising its impact. A spokesperson for MIND, a UK mental health charity, maintained that too frequently, mental health is referred to in relation to aggression and violence. He cautioned that, 'We must remember that there are 1.2 million people in touch with mental health services – and the overwhelming majority are not hurting others.' (Spokesperson for MIND quoted, in the *Sun* newspaper 7 October 2013).

De Angelis (2021, p. 3) points out that most violent acts are not owing to mental disorders, and that most people with such disorders are not violent. Also, when people with a mental disorder are violent, it often relates to 'contextual or background factors' like a history of childhood physical abuse and living in a poor district. Furthermore, factors predicting violence generally, such as antisocial behaviour and substance abuse also predict violence in people with a mental disorder (Ibid., p. 3).

Families and friends of victims killed by individuals with severe mental disorders including schizophrenia may want to convey the trauma of the homicide. One way of doing this is by ensuring that events are described in court and by the media without euphemism. In court, the victim's family and friends may feel side-lined. They may feel that comments from mental health charities and others are protective of people with mental disorder while minimising the shock and grief of those close to the victim. Such protective comments, instead of providing a context for the homicide, which is the intention, can be seen as one sided.

Guidance provided by the organisation A Hundred Families to note that, in courts of law, the proceedings often concentrate on the offender. Accordingly, defending lawyers usually present a range of reasons why the offender should be dealt leniently. This leads to the unfortunate consequence the organisation argues that 'The voice of the victim, and the impact their violent death has had on the family, can often be completely lost in this process' (A Hundred Families, 2015, p. 13, Practical Guidance).

Wehring and Carpenter (2011) recognised that, '... the field may have failed to adequately address violence.' One reason for this is owing to 'our eagerness to reduce stigma by emphasizing that persons with schizophrenia are more likely to be victims than perpetrators.'

Criticism of attributing stigma in schizophrenia to 'biological psychiatry' – misrepresenting biopsychosocial psychiatry as exclusively biological

'Biological' psychiatry

Critics reject the view that stigma is predominantly related to harm perpetrated by people with schizophrenia and the perceived risk of it. They tend to focus more on the negative effects of a predominantly biological and physical view of schizophrenia which they seek to equate with orthodox psychiatry.

To ague this point, dissenters depict orthodox psychiatry not as biopsychosocial, but as predominantly or exclusively biological. Reinforcing this characterisation are terms like 'biological psychiatry' or 'bio-genetic psychiatry.' Schizophrenia may be described as a purely 'biologically based illness' implying that psychological and social factors are not recognised.

Where research in biopsychosocial psychiatry examines factors like genetics, brain anomalies, and neurochemical action, the focus and the evidence will naturally be on physical and biological factors. However, this does not imply that the research takes place in a vacuum. It forms part of a wider framework which also considers psychological and social factors. Where critics can sometimes mislead, is where they present biological aspects of psychiatry as isolated from psychological and social aspects and seek to equate orthodox biopsychosocial psychiatry with this caricature of 'biological psychiatry.'

Critics' mistrust of drug companies

Read, Haslam and Magliano (2013) in discussing prejudice, stigma and schizophrenia announce their perspective in their book chapter sub-title 'the role of bio-genetic ideology.' Bio-genetic psychiatry is implicated, and it is viewed as an ideology. From this perspective, drug company websites are not to be trusted because they portray schizophrenia as a biologically based illness, or a 'debilitating disease.' Indeed, the authors maintain that the role of pharmaceutical companies in this situation is demonstrated by a study that looked at websites concerning schizophrenia and who paid for them. It showed that over a half of the websites about schizophrenia are funded by drug companies. Furthermore, the industry sponsored sites are, 'significantly more likely than other sites to portray "schizophrenia" as a biologically based illness' (Ibid., p. 160).

Read, Haslam and Magliano (2013) refer to a study 'emanating' from a World Psychiatric Association campaign that aimed to improve attitudes towards schizophrenia. It conveyed as 'sophisticated' and 'knowledgeable' the view that schizophrenia is a 'debilitating disease' caused mainly by a chemical imbalance. Read, Haslam and Magliano (2013) point out that the study was 'funded by drug company Eli Lilly' (Ibid., p. 159).

While having little time for pharmaceutical firms, dissenters also mistrust such company-sponsored psychiatrists if these clinicians consider lack of insight (anosognosia) as a symptom of schizophrenia. Read, Haslam and Magliano (2013 p. 160) refer to a 'drug-company-sponsored American psychiatrist.' This psychiatrist has 'gone so far as to claim' that anosognosia is a manifestation of schizophrenia and that has a biological cause (Ibid., p. 160). For dissenters, drug companies are implicated in teaching the public to view schizophrenia as an illness leading to more use of drugs and greater discrimination. Read, Haslam and Magliano (2013) depict the situation, as 'spending millions of dollars (largely by drug companies) to teach the public to think like biological psychiatrists.' For these authors, this has led to two outcomes, 'more discrimination and more drugs' (Ibid., p. 165).

Criticism that biogenetic causal beliefs engender negative attitudes, and psychosocial beliefs promote positive attitudes – weak evidence and polarised research

Mental health literacy and biological perspective

In seeking to destigmatise schizophrenia for the public, one approach is to emphasise that it is an illness, like any other physical ailment. Members of the wider community would not normally blame someone for having a disease like dementia or a brain tumour. Consequently, it would be unreasonable for them to blame someone for having schizophrenia. Read, Haslam and Magliano (2013) consider mental health 'literacy' as an example of a destigmatisation programme reflecting these views. Jorm (1997) is said to have envisaged mental health literacy as an opportunity. It could be used to educate the public about the psychiatric background of schizophrenia and its biological basis, and its treatment including by medication.

Read, Haslam and Magliano (2013) reject mental health literacy approaches. They suggest that Jorm and others see those who believe more in a social model of schizophrenia as experiencing mental health illiteracy. These authors align themselves with, the 'millions' of people who 'understand that bad things happening can drive us crazy' and who favour 'human' solutions to chemical ones. They believe that Jorm implies that all this mass of people are suffering from 'mental health illiteracy' and that he is not the only one to make such claims (Ibid., p. 159).

. Note that for Read, Haslam and Magliano (2013) there are 'millions' of people involved, that they do not just believe in a social model but 'understand' its correctness, and that they prefer humans over chemicals. Meanwhile, family members of people with schizophrenia 'sold' the illness view of schizophrenia through 'psych-education programmes' (Ibid., p. 160).

Attitude studies

Read, Haslam and Magliano (2013) itemise 22 correlational studies concerning 'mental health,' 'psychosis,' and 'schizophrenia.' These studies report associations between:

- causal beliefs (biogenetic or psychosocial) and
- attitudes (suggested by sematic differential choices like 'safe/dangerous') or desire for social distance (reflected in behavioural intention questionnaires with items like 'willingness to be friends with').

Also noted are 17 experimental studies involving manipulations. An example is showing a video of the same person but with different causal explanations to two different groups of respondents. These studies strongly associated biogenetic causal beliefs with negative attitudes, and psychosocial beliefs with positive attitudes (Ibid., pp. 160–166). Read, Haslam and Magliano (2013) suggest that 'In total, 52 of the 57 findings (91%) show that the vast expenditure of drug company and taxpayers' money on biologically oriented destigmatisation programmes is not evidence-based' (Ibid., p. 165).

However, 16 of the 22 correlational studies, and only 5 of the 17 experimental studies concerned schizophrenia specifically. Weakening the findings further, all the studies dealt with projected attitudes rather than real-life behaviour.

Also, studies giving volunteers a choice of whether mental disorders are owing to biological or psychosocial causes polarises the issue. A more rounded picture of causality would be to take account of biological, psychological, and social influences. For example, it is recognised that, it is not a few genes that contribute to the risk of developing schizophrenia, but rather there is a likelihood that variations in many genes do so. As reported by the National Library of Medicine (2018), 'In most cases, multiple genetic changes, each with a small effect, combine to increase the risk of developing the disorder.' Also, it is recognised that genetic changes can interact with environmental factors associated with increased schizophrenia risk. These include 'exposure to infections before birth' or 'severe stress during childhood' (National Library of Medicine, 2018).

Conclusion

Today, the term, 'stigma' carries with it mainly negative associations. In an orthodox view, stigma is associated with the incidence of comparatively rare violence perpetrated by people with schizophrenia. This includes evidence that individuals with the disorder are at an increased risk for perpetrating violence compared to members of the public.

Criminal records provide information about harm perpetrated by people with schizophrenia. But focusing on these can understate the prevalence of aggressive behaviour in schizophrenia. Also, it can insufficiently recognise the burden on families and professionals of caring for individuals and coping with such behaviours. Reports of high-profile acts of violence appear to have a negative impact on public perceptions of schizophrenia. Reiterating the rarity of harm perpetrated by people with schizophrenia does not diminish the impact on families and friends of victims killed by individuals with schizophrenia.

A dissenting view of the origins of stigma towards individuals with schizophrenia is that it can be created by orthodox psychiatry which critics in this context misleadingly depict as 'biological psychiatry.' Dissenters tend to mistrust the marketing and research and research funding of certain drug companies. They argue that metal health literacy as a destigmatising programme was too biologically orientated. Dissenters suspect that mental health literacy was taken as an opportunity to educate the public about the psychiatric background of schizophrenia and its biological basis, and its treatment including by medication.

Studies have been carried out looking at causal beliefs of mental disorder (biogenetic or psychosocial) and attitudes or desire for social distance. Relatedly, experimental studies have been reported that use for example responses to videos. These studies suggested an association between biogenetic causal beliefs with negative attitudes, and psychosocial beliefs with positive attitudes. However, little of the research related to schizophrenia, and all had the weakness of dealing with projected attitudes using questionnaires and similar rather than examining real life behaviour.

From a wider perspective, studies that present volunteers with a choice of mental disorder being owing to biological causes or to psychosocial causes polarise the causal factors. A more rounded picture of causality would be to take account of biological, psychological, and social influences.

Suggested further reading

Appelbaum, P. S. (2019) 'In Search of a New Paradigm for Research on Violence and Schizophrenia' *American Journal of Psychiatry* 176, 9, 677–679. https://ajp.psychiatryonline.org/doi/10.1176/appi.ajp.2019.19070678

Valle, R. (2020) 'Schizophrenia in ICD-11: Comparison of ICD-10 and DSM-5' *Journal of Psychiatry and Mental Health* 13, 2, 95–104. April-June 2020 (translated from the Spanish). https://www.elsevier.es/en-revista-revista-psiquiatria-salud-mental-486-articulo-schizophrenia-in-icd-11-comparison-icd-10-S2173505020300145

References

Angermeyer, M. C. and Matschinger, H. (1996) 'The effect of violent attacks by schizophrenic persons on the attitude of the public towards the mentally ill' *Social Science and Medicine* 43, 1721–1728. https://www.sciencedirect.com/science/article/abs/pii/S0277953696000652

Appelbaum, P. S. (2019) 'In search of a new paradigm for research on violence and schizophrenia' *American Journal of Psychiatry* 176, 9, 677–679. https://ajp.psychiatryonline.org/doi/10.1176/appi.ajp.2019.19070678

Canadian Health Services Research Foundation (2012) *Myth: Reframing Mental Illness as a 'Brain Disease' Reduces Stigma.* June, Ottawa, Canadian Health Services Research Foundation.

Cooke, A. (Ed.) (2017) *Understanding Psychosis and Schizophrenia: Why People Sometimes Hear Voices, Believe Things that Others Find Strange, or Appear Out of Touch with Reality, and What Can Help.* Canterbury, British Psychological Society Division of Clinical Psychology, Canterbury Christchurch University.

Crump, C., Sundquist, K., Winkleby, M. and Sundquist, J. (2013) 'Comorbidities and mortality in bipolar disorder: A Swedish national cohort study' *JAMA Psychiatry* 70, 9, 931–939.

Davies, J. (2013) *Cracked: Why Psychiatry Is Doing More Harm than Good.* London, Icon Books.

De Angelis, T. (2021) 'Mental illness and violence: Debunking myths, addressing realities' *CE Corner* 52, 3, 31. American Psychological Association. https://www.apa.org/education-career/ce/mental-illness-violence.pdf

Dilley, S. and Kemp, P. (2019) Alexander-Lewis Ranwell: The triple killer who was arrested twice BBC News 2 December 2019. https://www.bbc.co.uk/news/uk-england-devon-50591491

Falk, K. (2010) *Understanding Bipolar Disorder.* Liecester, UK, British Psycholgical Society.

Hsu, M.-C. and Tu, C.-H. (2014) 'Adult patients with schizophrenia using violence towards their parents: A phenomenological study of views and experiences of violence in parent-child dyads' *Journal of Advanced Nursing* 70, 2, 336–349. https://pubmed.ncbi.nlm.nih.gov/23855926/

A Hundred Families (2015) *A Practical Guide for Families after a Mental Health Homicide.* HundredFamilies.org. https://www.hundredfamilies.org/wp/wp-content/uploads/2015/12/HF_informationBrochure-web.pdf

Jorm, A. (1997) 'Mental health literacy' *British Journal of Psychiatry* 177, 396–401.

McGinty, E. E., Hendricks, A. K., Chosky, S. et al. (2016) 'Trends in the News Media Coverage of Mental Illness in the United States: 1995-2014' *Health Affairs* 35, 1121–1129.

Morris, S. (2019) 'Killer of three elderly Devon men found not guilty of murder due to insanity' *The Guardian* (2 December 2019). www.theguardian.com/uk-news/2019/dec/02/killer-of-three-elderly-devon-men-found-not-guilty-due-to-insanity

National Library of Medicine (2018) 'Schizophrenia'. https://medlineplus.gov/genetics/condition/schizophrenia/

Neha, A., Gandhi, S., Manjula, M. and Padmavathi, N. (2021) 'Caregiver's experiences of aggressive persons with schizophrenia' *Indian Journal of Psychological Medicine* 43, 1, 10–15.

Onwumere, J., Zhou, Z. and Kuipers, E. (2018) 'Informal caregiving relationships in psychosis: Reviewing the impact of patient violence on caregivers' *Frontiers in Psychology* 9, article 1530 September. https://www.frontiersin.org/articles/10.3389/fpsyg.2018.01530/full

Pembroke, L. R. (2012) *Self Harm: Perspectives from Personal Expereince*. London, Survivors Speak Out.

Rabun, J. and Boyer, S. (2009) 'Violence in schizophrenia: Risk factors and assessment' in Kasper, S. and Papadimitriou, G. N. (Eds.) *Schizophrenia: Biopsychosocial Approaches and Current Challenges*. London, Informa Healthcare. www.taylorfrancis.com/chapters/edit/10.3109/9781420080063-29/violence-schizophrenia-risk-factors-assessment-john-rabun-susan-boyer

Read, J., Haslam, N. and Magliano, L. (2013) 'Prejudice, stigma and "schizophrenia": The role of bio-genetic ideology' in Read, J. and Dillon, J. (Eds.) (2nd Edition) *Models of Madness: Psychological, Social and Biological Approaches to Psychosis*. London and New York, Routledge (pp. 157–177).

Spokesperson for MIND a UK mental health charity quoted, in the *Sun* newspaper, 7 October 2013.

TASS (2016) 'Nanny killing a child transferred from remand prison to mental ward' TASS, 10 March 2016. https://tass.com/society/861433

Torrey, E. F. (2019) (7th Edition) *Surviving Schizophrenia: A Family Manual*. New York and London, Harper Perennial.

United Nations Office on Drugs and Crime (2013) *Global Study on Homicide*. UNODC. www.unodc.org/documents/gsh/pdfs/2014_GLOBAL_HOMICIDE_BOOK_web.pdf

US Department of Health and Human Service (1999) *Report on Mental Health of the United States Surgeon General*. Washington, DC.

Valle, R. (2020) 'Schizophrenia in ICD-11: Comparison of ICD-10 and DSM-5' *Journal of Psychiatry and Mental Health* 13, 2, 95–104 (translated from the Spanish). https://www.elsevier.es/en-revista-revista-psiquiatria-salud-mental-486-articulo-schizophrenia-in-icd-11-comparison-icd-10-S2173505020300145

Wehring, H. J. and Carpenter, W. T. (2011) 'Violence and schizophrenia' *Schizophrenia Bulletin* 37, 5, 877–878. https://pubmed.ncbi.nlm.nih.gov/21860032/

Whiting, D., Gulati, G., Geddes, J. R. and Fazel, S. (2021) 'Association of schizophrenia spectrum disorders and violence perpetration in adults and adolescents from 15 countries a systematic review and meta-analysis' *JAMA Psychiatry* 79, 2, 120–132. https://jamanetwork.com/journals/jamapsychiatry/article-abstract/2787197

5

GENETICS AND SCHIZOPHRENIA

Introduction

In this chapter, I first summarise an orthodox position towards genetics research and schizophrenia. This points out that considerable progress has been made in understanding the role of genetics. For example, as contemporary research has replaced earlier notions of their being a single gene cause of schizophrenia, a much more complex picture has emerged. This understanding continues to be developed to the present day, aided by advances such as the findings of the Human Genome Project and new technology.

Despite such progress, challenges persist and are recognised in an orthodox view. One concerns the variability in the clinical manifestation of schizophrenia and the absence of a biomarker to compensate for the shortcomings in the demarcation of phenotypes. (An example of a biomarker is a gene that helps to identify a physiological or pathological process). An attempt to tackle the problem draws on endophenotypes. These seek to bridge the gap between the high-level presentation of symptoms and low-level genetic variability. The aim is to segment behavioural symptoms into more stable phenotypes with a clear genetic link.

A dissenting position regarding genetics and schizophrenia raises various criticisms. Each of which has its own limitations. Some dissenting critics refer, potentially misleadingly, to a genetic 'basis' of schizophrenia which may suggest an over inflated and isolated role for genetics. Dissenters may emphasise old studies indicating familial factors while underplaying the importance of more recent research like epigenetic

DOI: 10.4324/9781003413554-5

findings and genome-wide association studies (GWAS). Overstatement may be employed to bolster a weak position.

Dissenters may choose nebulous targets of criticism rather than specific people. Accordingly, individuals and groups are not identified and therefore are rendered unable to answer any unjustified accusations. Finally, critics may impute malign motivations to modern genetic research and those involved in it, raising the spectre of the holocaust and Nazi atrocities. Such implications are quite unsustainable.

Orthodox and dissenting positions

An orthodox position recognises that genetics has a role in explaining schizophrenia. But the interaction of genetic and environmental factors is important. Both pre-molecular and molecular genetic studies show that genes are 'a strong risk factor for schizophrenia.' Genome-wide association studies (GWAS) on schizophrenia have been replicated, with some reaching meta-analytic genome-wide significance. However, much is unknown about the etiopathogenesis of schizophrenia and the interactions between genotype and environment. Researchers advise caution about evidence regarding 'the size of the genetic contribution' in the aetiology of schizophrenia (Henriksen, Nordgaard and Jansson, 2017).

Contemporary theories of the causation of schizophrenia hold that genes do not directly cause the condition but increase susceptibility to 'developing the disease if the person is also exposed to specific environmental factors' (Torrey, 2019, p. 131). A combination of 'multiple genetic changes' each having a small effect, appear to increase the risk of developing schizophrenia. Among environmental factors interacting with genes to increase risk are exposure to infections before birth and severe childhood stress (National Library of Medicine, 2018).

In a dissenting position, it is maintained that 'mainstream psychiatry' considers the genetic basis of schizophrenia to be a 'proven fact.' Psychiatry is said to have an 'uncritical acceptance' of the conclusions of twin and adoption studies concerning schizophrenia. Believing that studies have established schizophrenia as a genetically based disorder, researchers have tried to identify genes 'for schizophrenia.' A concentration on genetic research is believed to 'divert attention' from social factors relating to schizophrenia (Joseph, 2013, p. 85). Attempts have been made to relate classifications in psychiatric guidance such as the *Diagnostic and Statistical Manual of Mental Disorders* (American Psychiatric Association, 2013) to 'biological markers.' These attempts are considered to have failed (Rose, 2019, p. 79). Nothing has been discovered about the 'genetic basis' of schizophrenia (Ibid., p. 107). Even where genes are implicated in schizophrenia, the picture is so complex that it is believed that 'nothing definitive can be said' (Davies, 2014, p. 134).

Progress in understanding genetics and schizophrenia, and continuing challenges

Progress in understanding genetics and schizophrenia

Understanding genetics in relation to schizophrenia has come a long way since geneticists believed that a particular gene or very small number of genes might be responsible for the disorder. GWAS and other contemporary research has moved genetics understanding forward from such early notions to a more complex understanding. Writing in 2017, Henriksen, Nordgaard and Jansson state, 'In the last decade, genetic research in schizophrenia has experienced a new dawn.' This the authors state has been instilled with renewed positive hope because of developments and advancement in statistical approaches and in technology (Ibid. p. 1).

Readers may recall that an allele is one of two or more versions of a DNA sequence at a certain genomic location. Genome-wide association studies (Henriksen, Nordgaard and Jansson, 2017) interrogate the genome for associations between common genomic variants (single nucleotide polymorphisms or SNPs) or loci, and schizophrenia. Specific allele variants of genes found more frequently in patients than controls, are taken to indicate a genetic association. One important study (Schizophrenia Working Group of the Psychiatric Genomics Consortium, 2014) combined available schizophrenia GWAS samples into a single analysis. It identified 128 independent schizophrenia associations, spanning 108 risk loci of genome-wide significance.

Polygenic traits are governed by multiple genes, and a substantial polygenic component of schizophrenia risk is found in thousands of common alleles, each having a tiny effect. Individually these do not attain significance. But cumulatively they may account for a quarter to a half of the variance in genetic liability (International Schizophrenia Consortium, Purcell et al., 2009). Henriksen, Nordgaard and Jansson (2017) similarly emphasises that the genetic architecture of schizophrenia is 'very complex, heterogeneous, and polygenic.' No matter how complicated and diverse in nature this is, it is hard to deny that it gives a more accurate picture than the notion that only one or two genes were implicated in schizophrenia.

There have been some false dawns in genetics research, leading to claims that great leaps forward were imminent. Refreshingly therefore, Henriksen, Nordgaard and Jansson (2017) give a considered summary of the position of modern genetics in relation to schizophrenia. They maintain that studies have demonstrated that genetics 'form a strong risk factor for schizophrenia.' Not only have many findings for GWAS schizophrenia studies been replicated, but several have 'reached meta-analytic genome-wide significance' (Ibid.). 'Robust associations' have been found between schizophrenia and more than 100 susceptibility loci. Identified copy number variations (CNVs) and single nucleotide variations (SNVs) 'seem promising' (Ibid.). The authors stress the importance of the thousands of alleles which, 'collectively form a substantial polygenic component of schizophrenia risk' (Ibid.).

Avramopoulos (2018) also recognises recent steps forward, maintaining that during the previous ten years, advancements in genetics has been impressive. Evidence cited for this view is that research previously had uncovered 'not a single known genetic risk variant or gene.' Failure to replicate previous research was normal. The author recognises that this was a 'difficult period for psychiatric genetics investigators' and maintains that the situation continues to affect the way that some commentators view the filed currently. The position today, is that researchers 'know of numerous robustly supported genetic variants' as well as CNVs. Also, there is robust evidence supporting the involvement of 'rare and de novo variants with stronger effects on the risk' (Ibid., p. 45).

Nevertheless, it is true that there are areas in which knowledge is still limited. These include the processes that initiate and maintain schizophrenia (etiopathogenesis) and the genotype-environment interactions for schizophrenia.

Challenges regarding phenotypic demarcation: endophenotypes and other responses

Challenges continue in the efforts to understand genetic aspects of schizophrenia. One concerns the difficulty in demarcating the characteristics of an individual with schizophrenia that have resulted from the interaction of their genotype with the environment (their phenotype). This is made difficult in the absence of a biomarker for schizophrenia, that is, in the present context, a gene or molecule that helps to identify a disease or pathological process. As Henriksen, Nordgaard and Jansson (2017) put it, a problem is the seeming variability in the 'clinical manifestation of schizophrenia' as well as the lack of, 'a biomarker to compensate for the shortcomings in phenotypic demarcation' (Ibid.).

One attempt to tackle the problem draws on endophenotypes which aim to bridge the gap between high-level symptom presentation and low-level genetic variability. An endophenotype (or intermediate phenotype) represents an attempt to segment behavioural symptoms into more stable phenotypes with a clear genetic link.

In schizophrenia, if psychosis is taken as a symptom, an underlying phenotype could be an impairment in working memory. Another such phenotype could be lack of sensory gating, a process of separating irrelevant and relevant stimuli, which in schizophrenia may affect associated cognitive deficits, and sensory overload. Both impairment in working memory and lack of sensory gating have a genetic component and can be seen as endophenotypes.

Work on endophenotypes may complement wide scale research like GWAS. In large samples required for GWAS, patients are typically grouped together by diagnosis and compared with control groups. With disorders like schizophrenia, which have diverse symptoms, genetic signals may be obscured (Greenwood et al., 2019). As biomarkers of underlying brain dysfunctions, endophenotypes might be able to focus on segments of the clinical symptoms of schizophrenia.

Endophenotypes can offer measures of specific neurobiological functions such as memory or inhibition. These have relevance for schizophrenia and are more objective than clinical symptoms. Where neurocognitive endophenotypes can be associated with real world functioning, this can be used as targets for developing treatment. For example, focused cognitive training can improve verbal memory in individuals with schizophrenia (Greenwood et al., 2019).

Baron (2001) identifies other attempts to circumvent this problem of shortcomings of phenotypic demarcation. One strategy is to dissect schizophrenia into clinical subtypes aggregating in families, for example 'periodic catatonia' (Ibid.). Readers may recall that catatonia is a 'marked psychomotor disturbance' involving decreased motor activity and decreased engagement, or 'excessive and peculiar' motor activity (American Psychiatric Association, 2013, p. 119). Another approach is to blur diagnostic boundaries between schizophrenia and other disorder. For example, some genetic findings indicate an overlap of genetic susceptibility loci between schizophrenia and bipolar disorder (Cross-Disorder Group of the Psychiatric Genomics Consortium, 2013).

Henriksen, Nordgaard and Jansson (2017) draw attention to some areas where caution is required. They recognise certain 'statistical facts' in schizophrenia. These include associations between common genetic variants (single nucleotide polymorphisms or SNPs) and uncommon genetic variants (copy number variations – CNVs, and single nucleotide variations – SNVs). However, these are not necessarily 'indicators of causal pathways.' Also, many of the associations that have been discovered are non-specific to schizophrenia and indicate genetic vulnerability to several mental disorders. Furthermore, details of the etiopathogenesis of schizophrenia and the genotype-environment interactions are still not known (Ibid.).

In short, contemporary genetics research can point to having developed greater understanding of the role of genetics in schizophrenia. It is also recognised that there are challenges in developing comprehension further. Outside of the constructive self-criticism generated by geneticists, which helps to drive research forward, there are dissenting views which tend not to engage with the latest findings and progress. It is to these that we now turn.

Dissenting views

Dissenting views about genetics and schizophrenia are various, and have weaknesses as criticisms. These are as follows:

- They refer loosely to a genetic 'basis' of schizophrenia
- They make a disputable emphasis when reviewing genetic research
- They employ overstatement
- They pick nebulous targets of criticism
- They impute malign motivations in genetic research which are unsubstantiated.

Referring loosely to a genetic basis of schizophrenia

In discussions of heritability and schizophrenia, it may be stated that 'studies suggest that schizophrenia is familial, and that genetic effects are the predominant model for its familiality' (Schosser and McGuffin, 2009, p. 84). Clinicians and others may question whether genes are solely a direct cause ('genes themselves do not cause the disease'). The role of genetics in increasing susceptibility to schizophrenia may be seen in relation to 'specific environmental factors' (Torrey, 2019, p. 131). Genes may be said to play a 'modest' role, and schizophrenia may be seen as 'not primarily a genetic disease' (Ibid., p. 133). Such comments reflect the view that interactions of genetic, lifestyle and environmental factors are embedded in modern considerations of the role of genetics (National Library of Medicine, 2021).

Despite such observations indicating the position of genetics in a biopsychosocial approach, the phrasing of criticisms of a possible genetic contribution to schizophrenia can be unclear. Some taking a dissenting position may refer to 'the genetic **basis** of schizophrenia' which 'mainstream psychiatry' is said to accept as an incontrovertible fact (Joseph, 2013, p. 85, bold added). Similarly, these critics refer to and reject the 'mistaken belief' that schizophrenia has been established as 'a genetically **based** disorder.' Relatedly, 'psychiatric molecular genetic researchers' have tried to find 'genes for schizophrenia' (Ibid., bold added).

Rose (2019) after summarising developments including in GWAS in schizophrenia, asks what has been established. He recognises the discovery of many small variations in basic neural processes. Each of these in different combinations, he notes, may bring about a small increase or decrease in the risk of a person being diagnosed with any one of many mental disorders. However, he rejects the idea that we have 'discovered anything about the genetic **basis**' of schizophrenia (Ibid., p. 107, bold added).

Rose (2019) accepts that for basic neuronal processes, there is evidence of a large number of variations among people. He further acknowledges that some of these are, 'linked to variations in inherited DNA.' But as to whether we have discovered anything regarding the 'genetic **basis**' of schizophrenia, Rose thinks not (Ibid., p. 107, bold added). Yet such view surely insufficiently recognises progress that has been made in understanding that genetic contribution is not simple and that it does not involve a single gene or a small number of genes having a direct effect.

Also, such criticisms present the difficulty of knowing exactly what is meant by schizophrenia having a 'genetic basis.' If the condition is genetically 'based' this may suggest that genetic contributions can act as it were on their own without interaction of other factors. Similarly, a genetic basis might imply that genes are foundational and more important than lifestyle or environmental influences. Such an implied centrality may not be accepted by orthodox practitioners, making criticism of this kind misplaced. To speak of a 'genetic basis' for schizophrenia seems to imply that there is a separable foundational genetic component rather than a complex interaction between genes and environmental influences. It makes no more sense than speaking of an environmental basis or a social basis for schizophrenia.

Finally, as a council of despair, dissenters may state that in schizophrenia, 'genes may be implicated' but the research is so complicated that 'nothing definitive can be said' (Davies, 2014, p. 134).

Disputable emphases when reviewing genetic research

Family, twin, and adoption studies constitute the early pre-molecular work on heritability and schizophrenia. Looking at work on twin studies may serve as examples of this sort of research. Cardno and Gottesman (2000) describe what they call, the 'basic intuition' behind twin studies. This involves first distinguishing between identical or monozygotic (MZ) twins sharing 100% of their genes and non-identical or dizygotic (DZ) twins sharing 50% of their genes. Given that twins share the environment in which they are raised, researchers proposed that higher concordance rates in MZ over DZ twins 'most likely' results from genetic similarity (Ibid.).

Citing earlier research (Cardno and Gottesman (2000) refer to estimates of concordance rates for schizophrenia. Those based on European twin studies from 1963 to 1987, they observe, show higher rates for MZ (48%) than for DZ twins (17%). European and Japanese studies from 1992 to 1999 similarly show higher MZ than DZ concordance rates (Ibid.). A meta-analysis of twin studies estimates the genetic liability to schizophrenia at 81% (with a 95% confidence interval of 73%–90%). Compared with this, shared environmental influences were estimated to be 11% (with a 95% confidence interval of 3%–19%) (Sullivan, Kendler and Neale, 2003).

However, contemporary researchers and others look at these old studies with caution. They emphasise that, 'everything that is familial is not necessarily genetic' (Torrey, 2019, p. 132). Twin studies may have been the 'bedrock' of genetic theories, but it is now realised that high estimates of heritability of schizophrenia (of 80% or more) 'have no foundation in fact' (Ibid.). It is noted that the design of so-called classical twin studies has been recognised as 'controversial' and remains so. The validity of this research has been often challenged.

It looks as though the 'intuition' underlying twin studies is straight-forward but it is not (Henriksen, Nordgaard and Jansson, 2017, pp. 4–5).

Despite the widespread orthodox recognition that earlier family, twin, and adoption studies have limitations, some critics of genetic studies emphasise these old and necessarily indirect genetic deductions as if they were the mainstay of current research. Their narrative seems to be that geneticists uncritically accept these earlier studies and misguided by them, have blindly gone on to pursue genetic foundations in later genome research.

While these older studies indicate familial factors, such research cannot show the extent to which they demonstrate heredity compared with more recent studies. Yet Joseph (2013) covers over 11 printed pages with reports of family, twin, and adoption studies. By comparison, only two pages concern more recent (e.g., GWAS) research for genes relating to schizophrenia.

This skewed picture of the bulk of the discussion is indicated by the chapter subheadings: family studies; twin studies, the equal environment assumption: the Achilles heel of the twin method, other twin studies; adoption studies, methodological problems, and selective placement: the Achilles heel of Adoption studies, Denmark, Oregon, and Finland and Sweden. As if to get rid of any doubt about the author's stance, the direct genetic discussion is headed, 'The fruitless search for schizophrenia genes.' A more recent presentation by Joseph (2023) of the perceived problems of molecular genetic research covers similar ground.

By contrast, Schosser and McGuffin (2009) in a book chapter consid-ering 'Genetic and epigenetic factors in schizophrenia' devote one page to 'family studies' and 'twin studies' and four pages to more recent genetic research. The latter covers predominantly GWAS and epigenetic studies. GWAS, they note, have become possible comparatively recently and allow 'hypothesis-free systematic screens of the whole genome.' Consequently, they supersede the need to select 'arbitrary candidate genes' which was frequently founded upon, 'uncertain theories about the aetiology of the disorder' (Ibid., p. 84).

Any criticism of genetic research into schizophrenia focusing on older genetic deductions from family, twin, and adoption studies rather than recent genetic findings is considerably weakened.

Negative depiction of genetic research – overstatement

Overstated terminology may be used in relation to nebulous targets of criticism. Strong language is more easily directed at vague targets rather than at particular people where it may be challenged as libellous. In this context, critics depict psychiatric molecular genetic research as 'massively plagued' by false positive results. Regarding schizophrenia and other psychiatric disorders, there has been a 'stunning and unexpected *failure*' in trying to find genes for them (Joseph, 2013, p. 84, italics in original). Uncritically accepting conclusions of schizophrenia twin and adoption researchers is 'an appalling development' in scientific research history (Joseph, 2013, p. 85). Also, there has been disregard of the 'massive flaws' associated with genetic research (Ibid.).

Overstatement can arise to convey the supposed rigidity of the views of present-day researchers. In a largely historical chapter, Read (2013) out-lines the work of pioneers Kraepelin and Bleuler, who first identified and then broadened various behaviours which they linked with the concept of schizophrenia. Read states that Kraepelin and Bleuler wanted to prove that these behaviours were the 'symptoms of a disease' but also that the disease was inherited. Looking at the families of patients identified, Bleuler found hereditary 'tainting' not only among 90% of the families, but also among 65% of people considered healthy. Speaking of Bleuler, Read (2013) somehow concludes that, 'Unlike genetic researchers of "schizo-phrenia" today ... he understood that "queer" parents having "queer" children proves nothing about genetics' (Ibid., p. 28).

Critics emphasise supposed rigid belief and absolute certainty to the point of overstatement, in referring to the work of researchers. Reference is made to the 'widespread but mistaken belief' that family, twin, and adoption research has 'established' that schizophrenia is a genetically based disorder. Based on this wrong belief, 'psychiatric molecular genetic researchers' have tried to identify genes for schizophrenia (Joseph, 2013, p. 83). Furthermore, the quest continues, based on researchers' 'belief that it is beyond question' that schizophrenia is a 'highly heritable' disorder (Ibid., p. 83).

The use of the term, 'belief' suggests faith rather than a testable hypothesis, so seeking to undermine any scientific motivation for the research. But does such research have to be based on an 'established' belief or one that is 'beyond question'? Could it not be guided by indications that there could be a genetic aspect to familial schizophrenia? Could some researchers hold the view that as Torrey (2019, p. 133) states, 'genes almost certainly play some role in the causation of schizophrenia' even though 'modest'? Could some researchers of today recognise familial influences as well as genetic ones? Practitioners of overstatement brush aside more nuanced positions so that they can castigate researchers for views that few may hold.

Criticising 'the discipline' – nebulous targets of criticism

Sometimes it is unclear at whom criticisms about genetic research and theories are aimed. It said that 'mainstream psychiatry' sees the genetic basis of schizophrenia as a proven fact; that 'psychiatry' has uncritically accepted the conclusions of schizophrenia twin and adoption researchers; and that 'the discipline' has failed to critically analyse its own research (Joseph, 2013, p. 85).

'Mainstream psychiatry,' 'psychiatry,' and 'the discipline,' are rather broad targets and people's views of what they are and what they represent are likely to vary. Who exactly do you question when you want to know what 'psychiatry' is saying? Points against genetic theories would be better made if directed towards individuals who could then, if they wished, confirm, or deny what they did or did not believe was a 'proven fact.' Where this is not done, criticism becomes targetless and therefore pointless.

A particular researcher or groups of researchers may produce weak findings. Specific peer reviewers may not be critical enough of such work. Certain editors and editorial boards may publish these studies. But instead of pointing to individuals, critics may use broad, generic terms to implicate all researchers and the totality of psychiatrists.

Similarly, and shamefully, where there is mention of 'eugenics' 'forced sterilisation' and 'mass murder' the broad expression 'biological psychiatry' is used to draw a parallel between Nazi psychiatrists and modern-day clinicians (Read and Masson, 2013). More is said about this in the next section.

Imputed (sometimes malign) motivations in genetic research

Where critics consider that social factors are important and may be being ignored by orthodox practitioners, they may question the motives of researchers. One motive imputed by critics of researchers focusing on genetic studies is that it, 'successfully diverts attention from the social factors.' These are supposedly the factors that in part lead to people behaving in ways associated with schizophrenia. It is also stated that, 'genetic theories aid the interests of the social and political elites' as well as those of the pharmaceutical industry. These interests, it is said, are to maintain the view that the source of 'psychological distress' is physical rather than being part of environmental settings, including political contexts (Joseph, 2013, p. 85).

Are genetic researchers motivated by diverting 'attention from the social factors?' Are they driven by theories which they hold because they 'aid the interests of the social and political elites,' and help 'the interests of the pharmaceutical industry'? If so, who are these researchers? And what do they have to say in response to critics about their supposed motives? A less contentious point might emerge from this sort of criticism. This is that where family, social, and political factors can be shown to be contributing causes of schizophrenia that attention should be paid to them. This would at least be more precise and practicable than attributing unproven motives to researchers.

There is a maxim that debaters have lost an argument as soon as they accuse opponents of being like Nazis. Motives attributed to researchers can be unpleasant. In a book chapter titled, 'Genetics, Eugenics, and the Mass Murder of Schizophrenics,' Read and Masson (2013, p. 34) discuss the atrocities of Nazi Germany. They reject the notion that what happened there is unconnected with the way that 'biological psychiatry operates today' (Ibid.). These events are said to illustrate themes evident in 'the history of the treatment of people considered mad.' Genetic theories gave the 'motivation, the rationale, and the camouflage' for the events that occurred (Ibid.).

Psychiatrists led the development of the theory 'that undesirable behaviour is genetically transmitted' that was used to justify 'compulsory sterilisation and mass murder.' These are the genetic theories that 'dominate psychiatry today' (Read and Masson, 2013, p. 34). Also, everyone working in mental health should be vigilant about, their failure to recognise the numerous ways in which people harm others. These include harm perpetrated by 'mental health workers themselves' (Read and Masson, 2013, p. 43).

In brief, Nazi atrocities bear on current biological psychiatry; genetic theories provided the motivation, rationale, and cover for atrocities; a theory that undesirable behaviour is genetically transmitted was implicated, and genetic theories still dominate contemporary psychiatry. So, what are the implications for genetic researchers today? Are the authors really saying that any of these researchers would want to justify 'compulsory sterilisation and mass murder'? If so which researchers? If not, why provide dots to be joined between modern genetic research and the holocaust?

Conclusion

Today, the genetic architecture of schizophrenia is recognised as complex, heterogeneous, and polygenic. Risk of disease is constituted by numerous common genetic variants of very small individual effects and by uncommon, highly penetrant genetic variants of larger effect.

Among still limited areas of understanding are the etiopathogenesis and genotype-environment interactions for schizophrenia. Variability in the clinical manifestation of schizophrenia and the absence of a biomarker to compensate for weak phenotypic demarcation continue to pose challenges. Responses to this situation include attempts to develop endophenotypes. Where these can be associated with real world functioning, it can inform targets for developing treatment.

Criticisms by those having a dissenting position are characterised by referring loosely to genetic basis of schizophrenia, making a disputable emphasis when reviewing genetic research, using overstatement, picking nebulous targets of criticism, and imputing groundless, sometimes malign motivations in genetic research.

In criticisms of genetic contributions to schizophrenia, terms like 'genetic basis' can suggest that genetic factors are foundational, can act solely, and overshadow lifestyle or environmental ones. This is contrary to the view of those seeing genetic and other factors as equally important.

Critics reviewing evidence of genetic factors in schizophrenia, may overemphasise the status of past family, twin, and adoption research. Suggesting that current genetic research is fruitlessly seeking a supposed schizophrenia gene, dissenters may deemphasise contemporary developments like those emerging from GWAS.

Overstatement includes referring to psychiatric molecular genetic research as being 'massively plagued' by false positive results, and using expressions like 'appalling developments,' and 'massive' flaws in genetic research. It can imply rigidity in the views of present-day genetic researchers, presenting them as being incapable of recognising the role of parenting rather than heredity in influencing children.

Criticism is sometimes aimed at nebulous targets, such as 'mainstream psychiatry' and 'the discipline,' rather than being directed at individuals who could counter allegations. Similarly, the expression 'biological psychiatry' is used to draw a parallel between Nazi doctors and modern-day psychiatrists.

For some critics, Nazi atrocities are linked to how biological psychiatry operates today. Genetic theories are said to have provided the motivation, rationale, and cover for what happened. A theory that undesirable behaviour is genetically transmitted was implicated. Also, genetic theories dominate modern psychiatry. Today's genetic researchers, it seems to be implied, are tainted by Nazi atrocities.

Suggested further reading

Henriksen, M. G., Nordgaard, J. and Jansson, L. B. (2017) 'Genetics of schizophrenia: Overview of methods, findings and limitations' *Frontiers of Human Neuroscience* 11, 322. https://research.regionh.dk/files/68915239/Henriksen_MG_Nordgaard_J_Jansson_LB_Genetics_2017.pdf

Joseph, J. (2023) *Schizophrenia and Genetics: The End of an Illusion*. New York and London, Routledge.

References

American Psychiatric Association (2013) *Diagnostic and Statistical Manual of Mental Disorders Fifth Edition (DSM-5)*. Washington DC, APA.

Avramopoulos, D. (2018) 'Recent advances in the genetics of schizophrenia' *Molecular Neuropsychiatry* 4, 35–51. https://www.karger.com/Article/Fulltext/488679

Baron, M. (2001) 'Genetics of schizophrenia and the new millennium: Progress and pitfalls' *American Journal of Human Genetics* 68, 299–312. www.sciencedirect.com/science/article/pii/S000292970764083X

Cardno, A. G. and Gottesman, I. I. (2000) 'Twin studies of schizophrenia: From bow-and-arrow concordances to star wars Mx and functional genomics' *American Journal of Medical Genetics* 97, 12–17. https://pubmed.ncbi.nlm.nih.gov/10813800/

Cross-Disorder Group of the Psychiatric Genomics Consortium (2013) 'Genetic relationship between five psychiatric disorders estimated from genome-wide SNPs' *Nature Genetics* 45, 984–994. https://pubmed.ncbi.nlm.nih.gov/23933821/

Davies, J. (2014) *Cracked: Why Psychiatry Is Doing More Harm than Good*. London, Icon Books.

Greenwood, T., Lazzeroni, L., Maihofer, A., Swerdlow, N., Calkins, M., Freedman, R., Green, M. F., Light, G., Nievergelt, C., Nuechterlein, K., Radant, A., Siever, L., Silverman, J., Stone, W., Sugar, C., Tsuang, D., Tsuang, M., Turetsky, B., Gur, R. and Braff, D. (2019) 'Genome-wide association of endophenotypes for schizophrenia from the consortium on the genetics of schizophrenia (COGS) study' *JAMA Psychiatry*. https://www.semanticscholar.org/paper/Genome-wide-Association-of-Endophenotypes-for-From-Greenwood-Lazzeroni/d0774290ad6b773b4d3d4cf5c78984e6431793b8

Henriksen, M. G., Nordgaard, J. and Jansson, L. B. (2017) 'Genetics of schizophrenia: Overview of methods, findings and limitations' *Frontiers of Human Neuroscience* 11, 322. https://research.regionh.dk/files/68915239/Henriksen_MG_Nordgaard_J_Jansson_LB_Genetics_2017.pdf

International Schizophrenia Consortium, Purcell, S. M., Wray, N. R., Stone, J. L., Visscher, P. M., O'Donovan, M. C., Sullivan, P. F. and Sklar, P. (2009) 'Common polygenic variation contributes to risk of schizophrenia and bipolar disorder' *Nature* 460, 748–752. https://pubmed.ncbi.nlm.nih.gov/ 19571811/

Joseph, J. (2013) '"Schizophrenia" and heredity: Why the emperor (still) has no genes' in Read, J. and Dillon, J. (Eds.) (2nd Edition) *Models of Madness: Psychological, Social and Biological Approaches to Psychosis*. London and New York, Routledge (pp. 72–89).

Joseph, J. (2023) *Schizophrenia and Genetics: The End of an Illusion*. New York and London, Routledge.

National Library of Medicine (2018) 'Schizophrenia' *National Library of Medicine*. Bethesda, Maryland. https://medlineplus.gov/genetics/condition/schizophrenia/# causes

National Library of Medicine (2021) 'What does it mean to have a genetic pre-disposition to a disease?' *National Library of Medicine*. Bethesda, Maryland. https://medlineplus.gov/genetics/understanding/mutationsanddisorders/ predisposition/

Read, J. (2013) 'The invention of 'schizophrenia': Kraepelin and Bleuler' in Read, J. and Dillon, J. (Eds.) (2nd Edition) *Models of Madness: Psychological, Social and Biological Approaches to Psychosis*. London and New York, Routledge (pp. 20–33).

Read, J. and Masson, J. (2013) 'Genetics, eugenics, and the mass murder of "Schizophrenics"' in Read, J. and Dillon, J. (Eds.) (2nd Edition) *Models of Madness: Psychological, Social and Biological Approaches to Psychosis*. London and New York, Routledge (pp. 34–46).

Rose, N. (2019) *Our Psychiatric Future: The Politics of Mental Health*. Medford, Mass, Polity Press.

Schizophrenia Working Group of the Psychiatric Genomics Consortium (2014) 'Biological insights from 108 schizophrenia-associated genetic loci' *Nature* 511, 7510, 421–427. https://pubmed.ncbi.nlm.nih.gov/25056061/

Schosser, A. and McGuffin, P. (2009) 'Genetic and epigenetic factors in schizo-phrenia' in Kasper, S. and Papadimitriou, G. N. (Eds.) (2nd Edition) *Schizophrenia: Biopsychosocial Approaches and Current Challenges* (Medical Psychiatry Series). New York and London, Informa Healthcare.

Sullivan, P. F., Kendler, K. S. and Neale, M. C. (2003) 'Schizophrenia as a complex trait: Evidence from a meta-analysis of twin studies' *Archives of General Psychiatry*. 60, 1187–1192. https://pubmed.ncbi.nlm.nih.gov/14662550/

Torrey, E. F. (2019) (7th Edition) *Surviving Schizophrenia: A Family Manual*. New York and London, Harper Perennial.

6

BRAIN ANOMALIES IN SCHIZOPHRENIA

Introduction

This chapter firstly summarise points emerging from orthodox and dissenting positions. These concern brain anomalies in some people with schizophrenia, and whether schizophrenia is a brain disorder. I discuss imaging techniques like computerised tomography (CT) or magnetic resonance imagery (MRI) scans which indicate structural and functional brain anomalies in people with schizophrenia. These have been studied through repeated assessments at different stages of the disorder. Structural deficits include reduced grey matter volume, and the disruption of the integrity of white matter. Among functional anomalies identified have been abnormal neural activity when people with schizophrenia engage in certain cognitive tasks for example involving long and short-term memory. Specific parts of the brain have been related to changes, such as enlargement of the lateral ventricles, and reduction of the hippocampus (located in the temporal lobe).

Next, the chapter examines criticisms of research into brain differences in people with schizophrenia which point to possible flaws in the studies involved. These include the low reliability of the construct of schizophrenia which may compromise research findings because the subjects involved in research can differ widely. Critics point out that large ventricles are not a specific cause of schizophrenia given that they appear in other conditions, like alcoholism. Also, dissenters argue that environmental factors like childhood trauma may contribute to the development of schizophrenia and may be associated with brain anomalies.

DOI: 10.4324/9781003413554-6

The chapter examines some weaknesses of these dissenting views. Critics may overstate evidence to argue that antipsychotic medication causes brain anomalies. For example, they may cite studies that 'suggest' such an association but report them as 'confirming' this view. Also sometimes overstated is the possible role of childhood trauma. Critics may offer a mistrustful presentation of evidence concerning the role of drug companies, and the credibility of drug funded research findings and associated researchers. In presenting evidence in this way, critics may suggest that such researchers are driven by ideology rather than scientific rigor. A laudatory presentation of selected supportive evidence may be given by dissenters, for example aspects of an MRI study associating antipsychotic drugs and changes in brain volume.

Orthodox and dissenting positions

In an orthodox position, schizophrenia is a 'disease of the brain' like multiple sclerosis. Supporting this view, researchers can measure structural and functional brain abnormalities in people with schizophrenia. Because these anomalies were described before antipsychotic drugs were introduced (in the 1950s) they, 'cannot be attributed to medication.' Consistent structural changes are enlarged ventricles and decreased grey matter volume (Torrey, 2019, p. 118). Schizophrenia is associated with structural and functional brain changes in 'prefrontal and medial temporal lobe regions.' These are implicated in respectively working memory and declarative memory (Karlsgodt, Sun and Cannon, 2010). Structural brain anomalies occur not only in schizophrenia, but also in other conditions including 'bipolar affective disorder, [and] recurrent depressive disorder ...' (White, Rickards and Zeeman, 2012, p. 1).

Turning to a dissenting position, structural and functional changes are recognised but are considered to have causes other than schizophrenia. For example, larger ventricles have been attributed to 'environmental factors' (Copolov and Crook, 2000, p. 109). One possible environmental cause is trauma, especially when experienced in childhood. Where people with schizophrenia have been, 'abused or neglected as children' it is believed that this could account for schizophrenia, mistakenly put down to brain disease. Another environmental factor that may cause ventricular enlargement and cerebral atrophy is antipsychotics (Read, 2013, pp. 67–68). It is argued that for those with a 'psychiatric diagnosis' and taking medication, the drugs are 'at the least a very significant cause' of brain changes compared with others without a diagnosis and not taking medication (Rose, 2019, p. 109).

Evidence for differences in brain structure and functioning in schizophrenia

Torrey (2019) highlights the continuing debate among researchers as to which parts of the brain are primarily affected in schizophrenia. As neuroimaging techniques have been developed, their use has improved understanding, allowing many brain areas to be studied simultaneously. Also, post-mortem tissue of individuals who had schizophrenia have become more available through so-called brain banks. What has become clear is that, in schizophrenia, a network of many parts of the brain are implicated (Ibid., pp. 127–128).

Various sources of evidence indicate the existence of brain anomalies in people with schizophrenia, from single research projects to the meta-analysis of many studies. Karlsgodt, Sun and Cannon (2010) note that schizophrenia is associated with alterations in brain structure and functioning. These include changes in the prefrontal lobe area involved in working memory, and the medial temporal lobe region implicated in declarative memory.

Such features are shown in imaging techniques. These enable repeated assessments to be made during both pre-onset and post-onset stages of schizophrenia and in 'critical periods of brain development.' Neuroimaging research suggests that schizophrenia involves 'disrupted neural connectivity' the sources of which are seemingly both genetic and environmental risk factors. These effect prenatal and adolescent brain development (Karlsgodt, Sun and Cannon, 2010, Introduction).

Structural brain deficits have been seen such as reduced volume of grey matter, and disruption of the integrity of white matter. These deficits may be progressive over the pre-onset phase and the early post onset period of schizophrenia. Abnormal neural activity has been shown by functional imaging techniques. These are evident when patients pursue cognitive tasks which engage short- and long-term memory, emotional processing, and decision making. Such abnormal neural activity has been noted across phases of schizophrenia (Karlsgodt, Sun and Cannon, 2010, Introduction).

Bogerts, Steiner and Bernstein (2009) note early studies that have used pneumoencephalography. In this radiographic technique, cerebrospinal fluid in brain ventricles is replaced with oxygen or air to form a contrast medium aiding brain examination. Such pneumoencephalography studies provided evidence for enlargements in the cortical sulci (deep fissures between cortical folds), and in the brain ventricles, particularly in patients with chronic schizophrenia (Ibid., p. 87). Later research has confirmed this with scans using CT or MRI.

CT as described by the National Institute of Biomedical Imaging and Bioengineering is a computerised imaging procedure using a narrow beam of x-rays aimed at a patient and quickly rotated around their body. This produces signals that are computer processed to generate cross-sectional tomographic images (slices) providing more detailed information than conventional x-rays. Successive slices collected by the machine's computer are digitally stacked together to form a three-dimensional image of the patient. Allowing easier identification of basic structures, this procedure also enables possible tumours or abnormalities to be spotted (www.nibib. nih.gov/science-education/science-topics/computed-tomography-ct).

MRI as described by the National Institute of Biomedical Imaging and Bioengineering is 'a non-invasive imaging technology' producing three dimensional detailed anatomical images. Implicating protons found in the water that makes up living tissues, this technology excites and detects change in the direction of the rotational axis of these protons. MRI is often used to detect disease, for diagnosis, and for treatment monitoring (www.nibib.nih. gov/ science-education/science-topics/magnetic-resonance-imaging-mri).

Giving 'convincing evidence' of changes are several meta-analytical reviews of structural imaging findings in schizophrenia. These are:

- enlargement of the lateral ventricles of about 30%
- reduction of the hippocampus by about 10%
- reduction of the temporal lobes by about 6%
- a subtle statistical decrease in whole brain volume of about 3%
- enlargement of the cortical sulci

(Bogerts, Steiner and Bernstein, 2009, p. 87)

In around a third of patients with schizophrenia, such changes are seen in routine CT scans or MRI scans. Where they are present, the changes vary from patient to patient, indicating 'considerable heterogeneity' in structural findings and in the symptoms and course of the condition (Bogerts, Steiner and Bernstein, 2009, p. 87). It is likely that schizophrenia, consists of an, 'inhomogeneous group of different neuropathologies and pathophysiologies resulting in similar clinical symptoms' (comparable for example to dementia and rheumatism). This might account for the very wide variance found in the neurological finding in patients with schizophrenia (Ibid.).

There is, 'Robust evidence from several replicated studies' showing prominent structural alterations in schizophrenia (Bogerts, Steiner and Bernstein, 2009, p. 87). These alterations have been identified in the limbic system (medial temporal lobe), the heteromodal association cortex, and the thalamus.

In the limbic system **medial temporal lobe alterations** involve the:

- hippocampal formation (located in the medial temporal lobe and involved in consolidating long-term memory)
- parahippocampal gyrus (situated along the ventromedial edge of the temporal lobe adjacent to the hippocampus and part of a region involved in memory encoding and retrieval)
- entorhinal cortex (a 'gateway' for information to and from the hippocampal formation contributing to the memory system and with a possible perceptual function), and
- amygdala (located in front of hippocampus and part of a neural system for processing fearful/threatening stimuli).

In the **heteromodal association cortex** (a region receiving input from multiple sensory of multimodal areas) are affected the:

- prefrontal cortex (the cerebral cortex covering the front part of the frontal lobe)
- cingulate cortex (located just above the corpus callosum on the medial side of the brain and an essential part of the limbic system)
- parietal cortex (the part of the cerebral cortex lying below the crown of the head)
- temporal cortex (mainly located in the middle cranial fossa, close to the skull base).

Structural alterations are also found in the **thalamus** (an egg-shaped mass of nuclei at the core of the diencephalon, which is a part of the forebrain). Its functions include relaying signals to the cerebral cortex, and regulating sleep, consciousness, and alertness (Bogerts, Steiner and Bernstein, 2009, p. 87).

Briefly then, imaging techniques like MRI and CT scans have indicated structural and functional anomalies in people with schizophrenia. These have been studied through repeated assessments at different stages of the disorder. Among structural deficits are reduced grey matter volume, and the disruption of white matter integrity. Functional anomalies include abnormal neural activity when people with schizophrenia engage in certain cognitive tasks such as those involving long and short-term memory.

Related to changes are specific parts of the brain. For example, lateral ventricular enlargement, and reduction of the hippocampus have been noted. Brain areas have been identified whose role suggests that anomalies could explain some features of schizophrenia. An example is the entorhinal cortex, a 'gateway' for information to and from the hippocampal formation. It contributes to the memory system and may have a perceptual function, which brain anomalies could affect. However, clinicians and researchers recognise that, among these findings, neurological observations vary considerably. These and other considerations lead to criticisms of research findings involving brain irregularities.

Why do the brain anomalies of larger ventricles and reduced brain volume tend to dominate debates between orthodox and dissenting positions? This may be because they are consistent and comparatively vivid findings which show up routinely in clinical scanning, becoming an agreed starting point for discussion. Also, ventricular enlargement and decreased cerebral volume seem to function as proxies in positions on whether brain anomalies are owing to schizophrenia as a brain disease or to other causes including antipsychotic medication and environmental factors.

Such is some of the evidence for differences in brain structure and functioning in schizophrenia. More speculatively, possible developments in the future have been put forward. Karlsgodt, Sun and Cannon (2010) consider the possibility of finding the molecular bases of changes associated with schizophrenia and their use in identification and treatment. Researchers could determine the molecular bases of the structural and functional changes associated with the disorder such as 'changes in neurotransmitter systems or cellular signalling' (Ibid., Conclusions). Then structural and functional changes indicated by magnetic resonance imagery (MRI) might be used to identify people with the greatest risk for the onset of schizophrenia. Treatments might be targeted at different subgroups of patients (Ibid.).

Dissenting views of brain anomalies in schizophrenia

Dissenters regarding brain anomalies and schizophrenia have raised issues relating to low reliability, lack of specificity of findings to schizophrenia, and the contribution of environmental influences.

- research findings may be compromised because the low reliability of the concept of schizophrenia may have led to the subjects of the studies differing considerably
- large ventricles being found in other conditions like alcoholism and depression, indicate that they are not a specific cause of schizophrenia
- environmental factors like childhood trauma may contribute to the development of schizophrenia and may be associated with brain anomalies.

Criticisms of research into brain differences in people with schizophrenia point to possible flaws in the studies. Read (2013) identifies issues arising when drawing conclusions about causation from brain research. For example, the low reliability (Read describes this as 'lack of reliability') about the concept of schizophrenia is identified as problematic. It raises the possibility that people studied by different researchers may differ markedly (Ibid., pp. 63–64).

An early study by Reveley (1985) found that between 6% and 60% of individuals with schizophrenia had enlarged ventricle ranges. Citing this, Read (2013) points out that because large ventricles are also found in other conditions such as alcoholism and depression, they cannot be said to be a specific cause of schizophrenia. He concludes that, all that is really known is that 'between 6% and 60% of people labelled "schizophrenic" have experienced one or more factors that cause enlarged ventricles' (Ibid., p. 67).

Environmental factors including childhood trauma may also have a part in the development of schizophrenia and may be associated with brain anomalies. Unidentified factors like trauma, especially in childhood when the brain is developing, may account for enlarged ventricles, rather than brain disease.

Some weaknesses of dissenting views of schizophrenia and brain anomalies

Some dissenting positions concerning brain irregularities have weaknesses. These involve:

- overstating evidence to support a view that antipsychotic medication causes brain anomalies
- overstating the possible role of childhood trauma
- mistrustful presentation of evidence concerning drug companies including their financial activities
- laudatory presentation of supportive evidence.

Overstating evidence that antipsychotics cause brain anomalies

Relevant to the role of antipsychotic medication in brain anomalies, is a review by Weinmann and Aderhold (2011) 'Antipsychotic medication, mortality and neurodegeneration: The need for more selective use and lower doses.' The authors searched medical literature to identify studies which assessed 'severe side effects of long-term antipsychotic treatment with a possible impact on mortality' and studies evaluating 'antipsychotic-associated brain changes.' This research found some evidence supporting reduction of frontal grey matter. Its authors carefully state that this reduction, 'seems to be accelerated by antipsychotic treatment and may depend on cumulative doses.' Also, the amount of the changes in brain volume was found to vary between individuals and according to the 'type and duration of antipsychotic treatment' (Ibid., bold added).

Also reviewing evidence, Navari and Dazan (2009) in 'Do antipsychotic drugs affect brain structure? A systematic and critical review of MRI findings' address two questions. These are, 'do antipsychotic medications induce changes in total or regional human brain volumes?' and 'do such effects depend on antipsychotic type?' This review found 33 studies reporting MRI measures directly in association with the use of antipsychotics and concerning, 'patients receiving lifetime treatment with antipsychotics in comparison with drug-naive patients or healthy controls.' The results concerning influence on the brain 'suggest that antipsychotics act regionally rather than globally.' Also, the changes in volume are greater when they involve the use of typical antipsychotics rather than atypical antipsychotics. There is evidence of typical antipsychotics specifically increasing the volume of basal ganglia structures. The study concludes that treatment using antipsychotics, 'potentially contributes to the brain structural changes' that are seen in psychosis. The authors express the view that future research should take note of 'these potential effects' (Ibid., bold added).

Citing the two papers just discussed, Read (2013) states that 'Recent reviews find numerous studies confirming that antipsychotics are related to reductions in brain volume and increases in ventricles' (Ibid., p. 68, bold added). But clearly, these reviews taken together do not 'confirm' this. Frontal grey matter reduction 'seems to be accelerated by antipsychotic treatment and may depend on cumulative doses' (Weinmann and Aderhold, 2011). Results 'suggest that antipsychotics act regionally ... on the brain' and antipsychotic treatment 'potentially contributes' to structural changes in the brain that are seen in psychosis (Navari and Dazan, 2009).

Read (2013) cites other research concerning antipsychotics and brain anomalies. Noting that others argue that the brain changes implicate not drugs but rather the disease process, he maintains that two recent developments have 'proved otherwise' (Ibid., p. 60, bold added).

One research paper concerns, 'The influence of chronic exposure to antipsychotic medications on brain size before and after tissue fixation: A comparison of haloperidol and olanzapine in macaque monkeys' (Dorph-Petersen et al., 2005). It reported on exposure to typical and atypical antipsychotics. The paper concludes that, 'chronic exposure of non-human primates to antipsychotics was associated with reduced brain volume.' Also, antipsychotics, 'may confound post-mortem studies and longitudinal imaging studies of subjects with schizophrenia that depend upon volumetric measures' (Ibid., bold added). The phrase 'associated with' is important. Clearly, the study does not claim to 'prove' that drugs rather than disease cause brain volume changes as Read (2013) seems to imply. Also inviting caution is that the study warns of possible confounding of post-mortem and MRI studies of people with schizophrenia, and that the research involves monkeys, not humans.

The second paper cited by Read (2013) was an MRI study by Ho et al. (2011) 'Long-term antipsychotic treatment and brain volumes: a longitudinal study of first-episode schizophrenia.' It looked at the study as it could be interpreted when considered alongside data from animal studies. The authors say that 'our study **suggests** that antipsychotics have a **subtle but measurable** influence on brain tissue loss over time.' They add that this influence on brain tissue can be taken as, '**suggesting** the importance of careful risk-benefit review.' Such a review would take account of dosage, duration of treatment, and the off-label use of antipsychotics (Ibid., bold added). Noticeably, the study 'suggests' a 'subtle but measurable influence' of antipsychotics, and 'suggests' a risk-benefit review in using medication. Again, Read, overstates the findings which, while raising issues, do not 'prove' his view (Ibid., p. 60).

Researchers clothe their findings in such circumspect terms for good reason. There may be several possible interpretations of the evidence of which the researchers have identified only one. They may want to see if other researchers replicate their findings so strengthening the evidence. If later research does not support the original findings, further studies may be carried out or the original interpretation of evidence may be revisited.

At the same time as describing tentative findings as cut and dried, dissenters may overlook arguments and evidence contrary to antipsychotics being related to brain anomalies. Abnormalities in the structure and function of the brain in individuals with schizophrenia, states Torrey (2019), were well described prior to the introduction of antipsychotic drugs in the 1950s. Consequently, anomalies cannot be attributed to medication (Ibid., p. 118). Some 20 years before the introduction of antipsychotics, a 1933 study reported that 25 of 60 individuals with schizophrenia had enlarged ventricles (Moore et al., 1933). This early evidence is supported by later research. Also, where studies involve patients with chronic schizophrenia who have taken antipsychotic medication, the relative contribution of the condition itself and that of antipsychotics is difficult to separate and distinguish.

Researchers have noted discrepancies in brain abnormalities between patients who are chronically ill and those in the early phase of schizophrenia. Reported especially in patients with chronic schizophrenia, brain anomalies are attributed to various possible factors. One proposal is that medication might increase brain abnormalities and could contribute to brain volume changes. Another possibility is that progression of the illness may lead to an increase of brain abnormalities.

Cahn, van Haren and Cahn (2009) note that for a long time it has been maintained that the changes in brain volume that are found in people with schizophrenia are in part caused by medication. However, they note that the decrease in brain volume may not be a 'direct effect' of antipsychotics. This is because, 'those who are prescribed the highest doses of antipsychotic medication are generally the most severely ill patients' (Ibid., p. 110). To look at it another way, where few brain abnormalities have been found in antipsychotic naïve patients with schizophrenia, this could relate to selection bias favouring the inclusion of patients with a less severe form of the disorder (Ibid., p. 107, paraphrased).

Overstating the possible role of childhood trauma

Evidence that trauma as an environmental factor may contribute to schizophrenia is debated. Torrey (2019) recognises that traumatic childhood events can leave 'lasting psychic scars.' He notes, 'Sexual abuse of children in particular has been plausibly linked to later depression, dissociative disorder, PTSD and substance abuse' (Ibid., p. 141). Also, a few scientifically sound childhood trauma studies report a correlation between trauma and the development of schizophrenia (e.g., Cohen, 2011).

However, weaknesses are identified in studies of childhood trauma and schizophrenia.

Suser and Widom (2012) point out that there is a central difficulty with research in this area. In nearly all studies, 'the measure of childhood adversity is weak.' It is also prone to bias, 'that could create an artifactual association with psychosis' (Ibid., p. 672). The authors note that nearly all the associations that are reported between childhood adversity and psychosis are dependent upon, 'retrospective recall of childhood adversity.' Can such recall, they ask, be relied upon to give 'unbiased estimates of association.' More broadly, doubt has been expressed for a long time in an 'extensive literature' regarding 'the validity of retrospective reports about childrearing, family conflicts, and psychological states in childhood' (Ibid.).

Read (2013) refers to schizophrenia and environmental influences. He cites identical twin studies where one has schizophrenia and larger ventricles and the other has neither (Copolov and Crook, 2000, p. 109). Read (2013) suggests that currently unidentified environmental factors may lead to increased ventricular volume, for example trauma, 'especially in childhood when the brain is developing' (Ibid., pp. 67–68).

However, Read (2013) then over reaches the evidence stating, 'Given that **the majority of people** diagnosed with "schizophrenia" had been **abused or neglected as children** ... this would account for much of the "evidence" that schizophrenia is a "brain disease"' (Ibid., pp. 67–68, bold added). He wants to reject that schizophrenia is a brain disease associated with larger brain ventricles, and to replace this with an environmental cause.

Questions arise from Read's (2013) claims. Where is the research that shows that 'the majority' of people with schizophrenia have been abused or neglected and how secure is it? What is the definition used to determine abuse? Is the abuse emotional, physical, sexual, or all of these? What is taken as 'neglect'? Are the reported accounts of abuse or neglect retrospective and if so, what is the assessment of their reliability? All these questions and more are side stepped in the phrase, 'Given that ...' But without such questions being addressed, the claim made by Read (2013) is overstated.

Mistrustful presentation of evidence concerning drug companies

In debates about brain anomalies in schizophrenia, critics may question drug company associated research. Sometimes this is done simply by pointing out drug company involvement without further evidence about the quality of the studies involved. It has been claimed that reviews find that 'numerous studies' confirm that antipsychotic medication is related to reduced brain volume and increased brain ventricles. Also, 'industry-sponsored studies sought to prove' that such findings applied to first-generation antipsychotic drugs, but not the newer atypical ones (Read, 2013, p. 68).

In an editorial, Lewis (2011) discusses 'Antipsychotic medication and brain volume: Do we have cause for concern?' This, Read (2013) disparagingly states, was written by someone 'who discloses income from eight drug companies' (Ibid., p. 69). In the editorial, mention is made of reductions in brain volume being beneficial in terms of reductions in cortical grey matter made in adolescence and accompanied by improvements in cognitive capacity. Read (2013) approvingly cites researchers who sarcastically suggest that Lewis is effectively saying, 'In other words, psychotic patients are hypothesised to have too much brain in the first place.' These researchers are said to be 'of a less ideological bent, and with no drug company sponsorship' (Ibid., p. 69).

Read (2013) discusses the findings of the MRI paper jointly authored by Ho et al. (2011). These findings, he says, were reported, attributed to researcher Nancy Andreasen, in the press three years before the MRI paper was published (*New York Times*, 2008). This seemingly means that 'Biological psychiatry and the pharmaceutical industry had three years to prepare their response to this proof that antipsychotics ... rather than the "illness" … is causing the brain atrophy' (Read, 2013, p. 69). Is it really being suggested that someone purposely allowed drug companies to prepare a response to the MRI study? Overstatement and conspiracy theory innuendo begins to replace rational argument and fair presentation of the evidence. Also, the vague terms, 'biological psychiatry' and 'the pharmaceutical industry' do not refer to particular people. Not identifying specific psychiatrists or drug company researchers, prevents such individuals from responding to the innuendo should they wish.

Laudatory presentation of supportive evidence

In contrast to mistrustful presentation of evidence concerning drug companies, aspects of the MRI study which associated antipsychotic drugs and brain volume (Ho et al., 2011) are conveyed in laudatory terms.

Pointing up perceived strengths of the research Read (2013) says, 'Not only did the study involve 674 brain scans, on 211 patients (**far more than most previous studies**) covering an average of 7.2 years (**the longest to date**), it controlled for substance abuse … .' (Ibid., p. 69, bold added). He describes the publication in which the article appeared as 'the **most prestigious psychiatry journal**.' The findings were announced to the press in September 2008 by Nancy Andreasen 'the **esteemed neuroscientist**' who is '**famous** for her separation of positive and negative symptoms' (Ibid., bold added). Prestige, esteem, and fame are of course appeals to authority and not relevant to arguments that the research is convincing or otherwise.

Conclusion

Regarding brain anomalies, early pneumoencephalography studies provided evidence for enlargements in the cortical sulci and brain ventricles, particularly in patients with chronic schizophrenia. This was confirmed by later studies using MRI or CT scans. Several reviews of structural imaging findings in schizophrenia indicate reductions in whole brain volume, temporal lobes, and hippocampus, and enlargement of the lateral ventricles and cortical sulci. Such changes are seen in around a third of patients with schizophrenia, and vary from patient to patient, indicating heterogeneity in structural findings and in the symptoms and course of the condition.

Prominent structural alterations are found in several areas. In the limbic system medial temporal lobe alterations involve the hippocampal formation, the parahippocampal gyrus, the entorhinal cortex, and the amygdala. In the heteromodal association cortex are affected the prefrontal cortex, cingulate cortex, parietal cortex, and temporal cortex. Structural alterations are also found in the thalamus. Schizophrenia likely comprises a varied group of different brain anomalies resulting in similar clinical symptoms, perhaps explaining the variance of neurological findings in patients.

Critics of research into brain differences found in people with schizophrenia point to the low reliability of the construct of schizophrenia. This may mean that people studied by one researcher may differ markedly from those investigated by another. Large ventricles do not constitute a specific cause of schizophrenia and are found in other conditions like alcoholism and depression. Brain differences do not necessarily indicate that they cause the symptoms of schizophrenia and might be brought about by aspects of the environment or external events.

Some dissenting views of schizophrenia and brain anomalies are weak. Critics may overstate evidence to support a view that antipsychotic medication causes brain anomalies. They may refer to reviews that are circumspect and cautious in 'suggesting' that antipsychotics could be related to reductions in brain volume and increases in ventricles. But in reporting them, they may claim that the studies 'confirm' such a finding. At the same time, a dissenting view may overlook arguments and evidence against antipsychotics being related to brain anomalies. For example, enlarged ventricles were reported in individuals with schizophrenia 20 years before antipsychotic medication was introduced. Also, brain volume decrease might not be a direct effect of antipsychotics as patients prescribed the highest doses are generally the most severely ill. Dissenters may overstate the possible role of childhood trauma in its contribution to schizophrenia.

Dissenters may offer a mistrustful presentation of evidence concerning the role of drug companies and dispute the credibility of drug funded research findings and associated researchers. Distrust of the role of drug companies can colour responses to research findings without any further evidence about the quality of studies. Critics may depict researchers with drug company sponsorship or who hold an orthodox view as ideologically motivated, evoking ridicule and innuendo.

Those holding a dissenting position may give a laudatory presentation of selected supportive evidence, for example aspects of an MRI study which associated antipsychotic drugs and changes in brain volume. This may valorise prestige and esteem over credibility.

Suggested further reading

Karlsgodt, K. H., Sun, D. and Cannon, T. D. (2010 August) 'Structural and functional brain abnormalities in schizophrenia' *Current Directions in Psychological Science* 19, 4, 226–231. https://www.ncbi.nlm.nih.gov/pmc/articles/PMC4235761/

Rose, N. (2019) *Our Psychiatric Future: The Politics of Mental Health* Cambridge. Polity Press.

References

Bogerts, B., Steiner, J. and Bernstein, H.-G. (2009) 'Brain abnormalities in schizophrenia' in Kasper, S. and Papadimitriou, G. N. (Eds.) (2nd Edition) *Schizophrenia: Biopsychosocial Approaches and Current Challenges* (Medical Psychiatry Series). New York and London, Informa Healthcare (pp. 87–104).

Cahn, K., van Haren, N. E. and Cahn, R. S. (2009) 'Imaging in schizophrenia' in Kasper, S. and Papadimitriou, G. N. (Eds.) (2nd Edition) *Schizophrenia: Biopsychosocial Approaches and Current Challenges* (Medical Psychiatry Series). New York and London, Informa Healthcare (pp. 105–113).

Cohen, P. (2011) 'Abuse in childhood and the risk for psychotic symptoms in later life' *American Journal of Psychiatry* 2011, 168, 7–8. https://ajp. psychiatryonline.org/doi/full/10.1176/appi.ajp.2010.10101513

Dorph-Petersen, K.-A., Pierri, J. N., Perel, J. M., Zhuoxin, S., Sampson, A. R. and Lewis, D. A. (2005) 'The influence of chronic exposure to antipsychotic medications on brain size before and after tissue fixation: A comparison of haloperidol and olanzapine in macaque monkeys' *Neuropsychopharmacology* 30, 9, 1649–1661. www.semanticscholar.org/paper/The-Influence-of-Chronic-Exposure-to-Antipsychotic-Dorph%E2%80%90Petersen-Pierri/f2f4af5c5a2c3942 66c37b9dd898ba1688607ad0

Ho, B-C., Andreasen, N., Ziebell, S., Pierson, R. and Magnotta, V. (2011) 'Long-term antipsychotic treatment and brain volumes: A longitudinal study of first-episode schizophrenia' *Archives of General Psychiatry* 68, 2, 128–137. https:// pubmed.ncbi.nlm.nih.gov/21300943/

Karlsgodt, K. H., Sun, D. and Cannon, T. D. (2010 August) 'Structural and functional brain abnormalities in schizophrenia' *Current Directions in Psychological Science* 19, 4, 226–231. https://www.ncbi.nlm.nih.gov/pmc/articles/PMC4235761/

Kasper, S. and Papadimitriou, G. N. (Eds.) (2009) (2nd Edition) *Schizophrenia: Biopsychosocial Approaches and Current Challenges* (Medical Psychiatry Series). New York and London, Informa Healthcare.

Lewis, D. (2011) 'Antipsychotic medication and brain volume: Do we have cause for concern?' *Archives of General Psychiatry* 68, 126–127 (Editorial 7 February 2011). https://www.researchgate.net/publication/49817142_Antipsychotic_ Medications_and_Brain_Volume_Do_We_Have_Cause_for_Concern

Moore, M. T., Nathan, D., Elliott, A. E. and Laubach, C. (1933) 'Encephalic studies in schizophrenia (dementia praecox): Report of sixty cases' *American Journal of Psychiatry* 89, 4, 801–810. https://ajp.psychiatryonline.org/doi/abs/ 10.1176/ajp.89.4.801

Navari, S. and Dazan, P. (2009) 'Do antipsychotic drugs affect brain structure? A systematic and critical review of MRI findings' *Psychological Medicine* 39, 1363–1377. https://pubmed.ncbi.nlm.nih.gov/19338710/

Read, J. (2013) 'Biological psychiatry's lost cause: The schizophrenic brain' in Read, J. and Dillon, J. (Eds.) (2nd Edition) *Models of Madness: Psychological, Social and Biological Approaches to Psychosis*. London and New York, Routledge (pp. 62–71).

Reveley, M. (1985) 'CT scans in schizophrenia' *British Journal of Psychiatry* 146, 367–371. www.cambridge.org/core/journals/the-british-journal-of-psychiatry/ article/abs/ct-scans-in-schizophrenia/51AD1594F27BE6A4576B6ACCE9339C0C

Rose, N. (2019) *Our Psychiatric Future: The Politics of Mental Health.* Cambridge, Polity Press.

Suser, E. and Widom, C. S. (2012) 'Still searching for lost truths about the bitter sorrows of childhood' *Schizophrenia Bulletin* 38, 4, 672–675. https://academic. oup.com/ schizophreniabulletin/article/38/4/672/1871240

Torrey, E. F. (2019) (7th Edition) *Surviving Schizophrenia: A Family Manual.* New York and London, Harper Perennial.

Weinmann, S. and Aderhold, V. (2011) 'Antipsychotic medication, mortality and neurodegeneration' *Psychosis* 2, 50–69. https://www.researchgate.net/publication/ 233138682_Antipsychotic_medication_mortality_and_neurodegeneration_The_ need_for_more_selective_use_and_lower_doses

White, P., Rickards, H. and Zeeman, A. (2012) 'Time to end the distinction between mental and neurological illnesses' *British Medical Journal* 344, e3, 4540. https://www.bmj.com/content/344/bmj.e3454

7
NEUROCHEMICAL FACTORS IN SCHIZOPHRENIA

Introduction

This chapter firstly looks at the 'original' dopamine hypothesis that excessively active dopamine transmission leads to the symptoms of schizophrenia. Research and theory concentrated on excess transmission at dopamine receptors and on treating psychosis by blocking these receptors. However, dopamine metabolites were found to be not universally elevated in the cerebrospinal fluid or serum of patients with schizophrenia, revealing a more complicated picture.

Version 2 of the hypothesis pointed to brain areas involving excessive or depleted dopamine transmission. It was proposed that overactivity of dopamine D2 receptor neurotransmission in the subcortical and limbic brain regions contributes to 'aberrant salience.' (Salience refers to the noticeability of stimuli, and aberrant salience concerns stimuli being given motivational notice so attracting attention and inappropriately effecting behaviour.) Aberrant salience manifested itself in positive symptoms of schizophrenia like hallucinations.

Negative and cognitive symptoms were attributed to underactivity of dopamine D1 receptor neurotransmission in the prefrontal cortex. But there was only limited direct evidence of elevated striatal dopamine function, and limited evidence of lower frontal levels of dopamine in schizophrenia.

Version 3 of the dopamine hypothesis offered a framework linking risk factors to increased presynaptic striatal (relating to the corpus striatum) dopaminergic function. These risk factors include genetics, pregnancy and

DOI: 10.4324/9781003413554-7

obstetric complications, stress and trauma, and drug use. Environmental stress and substance abuse interact with a genetic susceptibility, and lead to dopamine dysregulation. Increases in striatal presynaptic dopamine concentration cause psychosis or proneness to it through a process of aberrant salience to external stimuli.

Revisions to hypothesis 3 are envisaged leading to a stronger version 4. Future developments could include more information on the role of dopamine, particularly how genetic and environmental factors combine to influence the so-called common pathway, and the development of better drugs directly influencing presynaptic dopaminergic function.

Dissenting views have criticised the dopamine hypothesis and its related developments, but some of these are weakened for various reasons. The idea that the original dopamine hypothesis is still current and 'popular' overlooks the work that has gone into developments of the hypothesis over many years. A criticism that the original dopamine theory is simplistic and unsubstantiated is outdated as the hypothesis has been substantially developed. Claiming that researchers have continually failed to confirm the dopamine ('lead') hypothesis misunderstands or misinterprets the nature of hypotheses, which must be open to being refuted and modified leading to better hypotheses.

Where it is claimed that, after the 'failed' dopamine hypothesis, researchers turned to other neurochemicals this suggests a sequence of events that can be misleading. Where researchers recognised limitations in the earlier hypotheses and realised other neurochemicals had a role, as well as dopamine, it would be misleading to present this as driven by a 'failed' hypothesis.

A claim that most researchers envisage a purely chemical solution to schizophrenia is difficult to sustain. It cannot be assumed that even researchers focusing on genetic factors, because of the nature of the expertise and particular research, do not recognise environmental and other factors.

Critics may claim that 'failed' neurochemical explanations undermine justifications for using antipsychotics, calling into question the marketing of pharmaceutical companies basing their drug promotion solely on a claimed effect on the earlier proposed simple dopamine dysregulation. However, the hypotheses about dopamine have not 'failed' but have been modified and developed, and the action of drugs on dopamine and other neurochemicals also continues to be developed.

Orthodox and dissenting positions

A central hypothesis about schizophrenia and psychosis generally involves the neurotransmitter dopamine (produced in the mid-brain) and mechanisms relating to it.

This hypothesis has had a long history and has been adapted according to new evidence.

At first, dopamine was thought to be 'a precursor molecule of little functional significance.'

However, researchers have developed the idea, leading to an 'increasingly sophisticated account of the involvement of dopamine in schizophrenia' (Howes and Kapur, 2009, p. 549). Supporting the role of dopamine is that the 'mechanism of every effective antipsychotic medication' that is used to treat schizophrenia involves dopamine and its interaction with other neurochemical pathways. These interactions include those with glutamate, GABA, serotonin, and acetylcholine (Brisch et al., 2014). It is expected that continuing research will provide further information of dopamine's role, especially how 'genetic and environmental factors combine to influence the common pathway.' Also, it is anticipated that more effective medication will be developed, directly effecting 'presynaptic dopaminergic function' (Howes and Kapur, 2009, p. 557). Links are also found between dopamine functioning and some environmental factors associated with schizophrenia. For example, 'Measures of presynaptic dopamine function are raised in migrants, and those that have experienced childhood trauma' (McCutcheon, Krystal, and Howes, 2020, p. 25).

A dissenting position tends to focus on the first or early iterations of the dopamine hypothesis as if it had not been modified. It is stated that 'Biological psychiatry's lead theory of schizophrenia, for the past 40 years, is that it is caused by too much dopamine' (Read, 2013, p. 64). The original dopamine theory is described as, 'simplistic, and unsubstantiated' and still 'very popular.' It is said to be 'the cornerstone' of a claim in 'biological psychiatry' that schizophrenia is an illness. Furthermore, the theory supports marketing of antipsychotic medication by pharmaceutical companies. It is said that there has been a 'continued failure' to confirm the dopamine theory. This failure has led to researchers investigating the roles of other neurotransmitters like glutamate, gamma-aminobutyric acid (GABA), and acetyl choline (Ibid., p. 66).

Dopamine

Dopamine and its pathways: mesolimbic, mesocortical, nigrostriatal, tuberoinfundibular

Recall that a neuron is an electrically excitable cell communicating with other cells via special connections (synapses) and typically comprising a cell body from which extend filaments (dendrites and a single axon). At the tip of the axon (the axon terminal) the neuron can transmit a signal to another cell across a synapse. At the synapse, the plasma membrane of the neuron passing the signal (the presynaptic neuron) closely approaches the membrane of the target cell (the postsynaptic cell). Molecular processes link the two membranes and carry out the signalling process. Neurotransmission involves a brain cell releasing a neurochemical into the space between neurons at the synapse (synaptic cleft) and then binding with a receptor (a receiving cell). The neurotransmitter dopamine is produced in the mid brain, specifically in the ventral tegmental area and the adjacent substantia nigra.

Projecting from the ventral tegmental area (VTA) are two prominent efferent nerve fibres (carrying impulses outwards from the central nervous system). These two are the mesolimbic pathway which goes to the limbic area, and the mesocortical pathway travelling to the cortical area. The VTA, concerned with cognitive and emotional processes, appears to have a role in motivation, and reward.

The substantia nigra (Latin for black substance) is so called because it appears darker than surrounding areas owing to high levels of neuromelanin in dopamine related neurons. From it, fibres of the nigrostriatal pathway project to the striatum (caudate and putamen) a cluster of neurons in the forebrain (the subcortical basal ganglia) forming part of reward and motor systems. The substantia nigra is associated particularly with movement.

Also, dopamine neurons act in the so-called tuberoinfundibular pathway implicating the hypothalamus located at the base of the brain and having a role in several important functions including regulating emotional responses and releasing hormones. The tuberoinfundibular pathway projects from the arcuate nucleus of the hypothalamus (the 'tuberal region') and extends to the median eminence parts of the hypothalamus.

Essentially, the four pathways, mesolimbic, mesocortical, nigrostriatal, and tuberoinfundibular, are neuronal connections allowing dopamine to pass on information such as cognition, executive thinking, voluntary motor movements, and feelings of pleasure and reward.

Dopamine receptors

Dopamine receptors are expressed in the central nervous system (hippocampal dentate gyrus and subventricular zone) and in the periphery, including the kidney. Each of the five types of dopamine receptors D1 through D5 have various functions, some overlapping, and broadly identified as follows:

D1: memory, attention, impulse control, regulation of renal function, locomotion

D2: locomotion, attention, sleep, memory, learning

D3: cognition, impulse control, attention, sleep

D4: cognition, impulse control, attention, sleep

D5: decision making, cognition, attention, renin secretion (Bhatia, Lenchner and Saadabadi, 2021).

Other neurotransmitters implicated in refinements of dopamine hypotheses

Among other neurotransmitters implicated in the evolving dopamine hypotheses are

- glutamate
- gamma-aminobutyric acid (GABA)
- acetyl choline, and
- serotonin.

Glutamate is an excitatory brain neurotransmitter. It has been proposed that schizophrenia symptoms are owing to hypofunction of N-methyl-D-aspartate receptors (NMDARs) and excessive glutamate release, especially the prefrontal cortex and hippocampus. (Recall that the hippocampus is in the medial region of the temporal lobe. It is part of the limbic system which regulates emotional responses and is thought to help store and consolidate long-term memories, and to be involved in spatial processing.) NMDAR is a glutamate receptor and ion channel found in neurons. Supporting this that NMDAR antagonists (which interfere with the physiological action of NMDRs) uniquely reproduce both positive and negative symptoms of schizophrenia and induce schizophrenia-like cognitive deficits.

Gamma-aminobutyric acid (GABA) is a neurotransmitter inhibiting certain brain signals which decreases activity in the nervous system. When it attaches to a protein so-called GABA receptor, this produces a calming effect, helping people to manage feelings of anxiety fear and stress. GABA and glutamate act in opposite ways and a balance is maintained between the inhibitory effects of GABA and the excitatory effects of glutamate.

Acetylcholine is a neurotransmitter at the neuromuscular junction, being the chemical that motor neurones of the nervous system release to activate muscles. Parts of the body using or affected by acetylcholine are so-called 'cholinergic.' Substances increasing or decreasing the overall activity of the cholinergic system are designated cholinergics and anticholinergics respectively. Acetylcholine is also a neurotransmitter in the autonomic nervous system. It is an internal transmitter for the sympathetic nervous system and is the final product released by the parasympathetic nervous system. Various cholinergic areas of the brain each have distinct functions such as involvement in arousal, attention, memory, and motivation. Drugs affecting cholinergic systems can cause paralysis and convulsions.

Serotonin (5-hydroxytryptamine) has been implicated in behaviours and bodily functions disturbed in schizophrenia such as perception, attention, mood, aggression, and movement. Many substances blocking serotonin receptors have been evaluated for the treatment of schizophrenia. Clozapine having a high affinity for serotonin receptors has been found effective in treatment-resistant schizophrenia (Yamada, 2022).

Stahl (2018) focusing on hallucinations and delusions, suggests three interconnected pathways theoretically linked to these and implicating dopamine, glutamate, and serotonin.

These are:

- dopamine hyperactivity at D2 dopamine receptors in the mesolimbic pathway, extending from the ventral tegmental area to the ventral striatum
- glutamate theory of psychosis (the N-methyl-d-aspartate or NMDA hypoactivity theory) proposing that NMDA receptor hypofunction in the prefrontal cortex can result in psychosis
- serotonin hyperactivity at 5-HT2A receptors on glutamate neurons in the cerebral cortex.

Stahl (2018) notes that all three neuronal networks and neurotransmitters are linked. Also, both 5HT2A and NMDA receptor actions 'can result in hyperactivity of the downstream mesolimbic dopamine pathway' (Ibid.).

The development of dopamine hypotheses

Having considered dopamine and its pathways and receptors, and other neurotransmitters implicated in refinements of dopamine hypotheses, we can discuss the development of the dopamine hypotheses themselves.

Hypotheses of the role of dopamine in schizophrenia have passed through several iterations. Clearly what is understood today about dopamine, its pathways, receptors, and roles was not when the original hypothesis was framed. I am indebted in the following summary of versions of the dopamine hypotheses to the article by Howes and Kapur (2009).

Version 1

An early 'original' dopamine hypothesis was that excessively active dopamine transmission leads to the schizophrenia symptoms. In seeming support of this, was that psychostimulant drugs amphetamines can produce schizophrenia-like symptoms. Their action includes inhibiting the reuptake of dopamine by interacting with the dopamine transporter so increasing dopamine in the synaptic cleft.

In the 1970s, it was recognised that the effectiveness of antipsychotics related to their affinity for dopamine receptors. Research and theory concentrated on excess transmission at dopamine receptors and on treating psychosis by blocking the receptors. Accordingly, version 1 of the hypothesis emphasised the role of excess dopamine in the causation of schizophrenia.

Problematic for 'version 1' was that dopamine metabolites (products of dopamine metabolism) were not universally elevated in the cerebrospinal fluid or serum of patients with schizophrenia. Post-mortem studies of D2 receptors in schizophrenia could not exclude the potential influence of previous antipsychotic treatment. Furthermore, results of early positron emission tomography (PET) studies of D2 and D3 receptors in drug-naive patients were conflicting.

A more complicated picture began to emerge. Positive symptoms of schizophrenia were associated with subcortical release of dopamine which augments activation of the dopamine D2 receptor. Negative symptoms of schizophrenia were associated with reduced activation of the dopamine D1 receptor in the prefrontal cortex and decreased activity of the nucleus caudatus (part of the corpus striatum structure).

Version 2

Accordingly, Davis et al. (1991) reconceptualized the dopamine hypothesis recognising that dopamine receptors show different brain distributions. It was proposed that overactivity of the dopamine D2 receptor neurotransmission in subcortical and limbic brain regions contributes to a faulty emphasis being placed on some external stimuli. This 'aberrant salience' manifested itself in positive symptoms of schizophrenia like hallucinations. Negative and cognitive symptoms could be attributed to underactivity of dopamine D1 receptor neurotransmission in the pre-frontal cortex.

However, much of the supporting evidence for this hypothesis relied on inferences from animal studies or from other clinical conditions. Direct evidence for low dopamine levels in the frontal cortex was lacking. Only limited direct evidence indicated elevated striatal dopamine function. (Striatal dopamine release involves mechanisms driving activity in mid-brain dopamine neurons and mechanisms in the striatum that act on and within dopamine axons.) It was unclear how the dopamine abnormalities were linked to clinical features.

Gradually it emerged that the cortical abnormalities were more complicated than originally thought. Also, there was limited evidence of lower frontal levels of dopamine in schizophrenia. Version 2 of the theory did not describe the etiological origins of the dopamine related abnormality, nor pinpoint which element of dopamine transmission was abnormal.

Version 3

Howes and Kapur (2009) reviewed data to identify new evidence in neurochemical imaging studies, genetic evidence, findings on environmental risk factors, research into the extended phenotype, and animal studies. Developing a version 3 of the dopamine hypothesis, they called it 'the final common pathway.' This offered a framework linking risk factors to increased presynaptic striatal dopaminergic function. These risk factors include genetics, pregnancy and obstetric complications, stress and trauma, and drug use.

Furthermore, the hypothesis accounts for a complex range of findings like frontotemporal structural and functional abnormalities, and cognitive impairments. It explains how these may converge neurochemically to cause psychosis through aberrant salience leading to a diagnosis of schizophrenia. Because current treatments are acting 'downstream' of the critical neurotransmitter abnormality, the hypothesis proposes that future drug research focuses on identifying and manipulating 'upstream' factors that converge on the dopaminergic funnel point.

Briefly, version 3 proposes that environmental stress and substance abuse interact with a genetic susceptibility, and lead to dopamine dysregulation. Increases in striatal presynaptic dopamine concentration cause psychosis or proneness to it through a process of aberrant salience to external stimuli.

Towards version 4?

Howes and Kapur (2009, pp. 556–557) identify the two main claims of version 3: that the presynaptic abnormality is primary, and that dopamine is the final common pathway.

Two kinds of evidence could contradict this.

Firstly, PET studies directly implicating presynaptic dopamine dysfunction are crucial. PET data must be modelled to give estimates of L-dopa uptake or synaptic dopamine levels, the results being inferred, not direct measurements. Therefore, it would damage version 3 if the validity of PET imaging was compromised. This could arise if evidence was found to be a 'confound' of modelling or technical approaches (an additional variable discovered to be related to both predictors and outcomes). This would compromise internal validity by making researchers unable to tell whether the outcome is caused by the predictor or the confounding variable. Also damaging is if evidence is discovered to be an artifact of modelling and technical approaches. This could mean that study findings apply only to the specific situation tested, threatening external validity because it may not be possible to generalise results from the population of the study.

Another threat would be the discovery of a new drug that treats psychosis without a direct effect on the dopamine system, so that dopamine abnormalities continue unabated, despite psychosis being reduced. Also problematic for version 3 would be if a pathophysiological mechanism not impacting the dopamine system is found to be universal to schizophrenia. More likely is that the hypothesis will be revised into a stronger version 4.

Continuing research

Juar and colleagues (2017) examined the role of striatal dopamine synthesis capacity in patients with bipolar disorders with a current or previous psychotic episode, compared with patients with first-episode schizophrenia and with healthy controls. They tested the transdiagnostic dopamine hypothesis of psychosis using PET imaging to examine bipolar affective disorder and schizophrenia. 'Transdiagnostic' implies that dopamine abnormalities underlie psychosis, irrespective of diagnosis.

Juar and colleagues (2017) found that striatal dopamine synthesis capacity:

- was significantly elevated in both bipolar and schizophrenia group compared with controls
- showed no significant difference between the bipolar and schizophrenia group
- was significantly positively correlated with positive psychotic symptom severity in the combined bipolar and schizophrenia sample experiencing a current psychotic episode, and
- was significantly positively associated with positive psychotic symptom severity in individuals with bipolar disorder experiencing a current psychotic episode, even allowing for manic symptom severity.

These findings were consistent with a transdiagnostic role for dopamine dysfunction in the development of psychosis, suggesting that dopamine synthesis capacity could be a potential novel drug target for bipolar disorder and schizophrenia.

Referring to the study by Juar and colleagues (2017) and issues arising, Hengartner and Moncrieff (2018) suggest that evidence supporting version 3 is 'inconclusive.' They identify several difficulties relating to:

- the effect of previously taken antipsychotic medication
- the potential confounding of results by stress and substance abuse
- statistical issues relating to few participants, and
- potential bias involved in comparing healthy controls with inpatients having schizophrenia.

For example, comparing healthy controls to inpatients with schizophrenia can create bias. These groups may differ regarding childhood adversity, socio-economic status, lifestyle, and physical health. But dopamine research typically matches controls to inpatients based on sex, age, and ethnicity only. Better would be to contrast patients with schizophrenia with equally distressed but non-psychotic patients, who unlike healthy controls may be more comparable in personal history of adversity, psychosocial impairments, and current levels of acute arousal and stress.

Howes and Kapur (2009) believe that hypothesis 3 is likely to be revised, 'with a stronger version IV.' They expect future developments to include more information on the role of dopamine, particularly how genetic and environmental factors combine to influence the common pathway, and better drugs that directly influence presynaptic dopaminergic function (Ibid., pp. 556–557). We now turn to criticisms of dopamine theory which sometimes touch on neurochemical perspectives of schizophrenia more broadly.

Dissenting criticisms

Dissenting views relating to the dopamine hypotheses tend to cleave to an out-of-date position that the original dopamine hypothesis is still current, ignoring its later iterations. This allow critics to state that the hypothesis is 'simplistic' and has 'failed.' The supposed failure leads to claims that this precipitated work on other neurochemical, and that it undermines justifications for administering antipsychotics.

This is reflected in the areas discussed below that:

- the original dopamine hypothesis is still current and 'popular'
- the original dopamine theory is simplistic and unsubstantiated
- researchers have continually failed to confirm the dopamine ('lead') hypothesis

- after the failed dopamine hypothesis, researchers turned to other neurochemicals
- orthodox researchers envisage a purely chemical 'solution' to schizophrenia
- 'failed' neurochemical explanations undermine justifications for using antipsychotics.

The original dopamine hypothesis is still current and 'popular'

Critics have stated that 'Biological psychiatry's lead theory of schizophrenia, for the past 40 years, is that it is caused by too much dopamine' (Read, 2013, p. 64). However, the present tense in this expression misleads. A 'too much dopamine' hypothesis was the original version of a theory in the light of evidence available at the time.

As we have seen the hypothesis evolved according to new evidence and in relation to new technology and procedures. However, critics maintain that the early theory remains 'very popular' (Read, 2013, p. 64) but whatever, 'very popular' might mean in this context, this surely cannot apply to the researchers who developed later versions or others who are aware of refinements to the theory introduced in later iterations.

The original dopamine theory is simplistic and unsubstantiated

As already touched on, it is remarked that, '… the original, simplistic, and unsubstantiated dopamine theory remains very popular' (Read, 2013, p. 66). Anything that is 'simplistic' rather than 'simple' in the positive sense is unlikely to be useful. It follows that the description of the early theory as 'simplistic' conveys a rejection of it. However, this description is surely outdated.

The early theory was based on then current evidence and as new information emerged, it was found that in trying to cover schizophrenia as an entity, the hypothesis was too broad. If the theory was found to be 'unsubstantiated' as new evidence became available, this is surely a strength showing that it could be further developed or shown to be wanting and dispensed with.

Researchers have continually failed to confirm the dopamine ('lead') hypothesis

To speak of the 'continued failure to confirm biological psychiatry's lead hypothesis' (Read, 2013, p. 66) is to misrepresent the nature of hypotheses in general and the dopamine hypotheses particularly. Good hypotheses are by their nature amenable to being confirmed (always provisionally) or disconfirmed. They can also be confirmed in certain aspects and not in others, leading to further refinements.

After the failed dopamine hypothesis, researchers turned to other neurochemicals

Another observation is that the supposed persisting 'failure' to 'confirm biological psychiatry's lead hypothesis led to the investigation of other neurotransmitters ...' (Read, 2013, p. 66). If it is accepted that confirmation of the dopamine hypothesis did not 'fail,' but pointed to refinements, it is misleading to suggest that this 'led to' researchers turning to other neurotransmitters. In fact, the dopamine hypothesis continued and continues to be developed.

Research into other neurotransmitters also continues, including the ways that these interact with dopamine. In examining the role of dopamine in schizophrenia 'from a neurobiological and evolutionary perspective,' Brisch and colleagues (2014) include a section on 'alternative neurochemical models in schizophrenia and their interaction with dopamine' discussing the relationships between dopamine and other neurochemicals. These authors also note, '... to date, the mechanism of every effective antipsychotic medication in schizophrenia involves dopamine and its interaction with other neurochemical pathways such as those of glutamate, GABA, serotonin, and acetylcholine' (Ibid.).

Orthodox researchers envisage a purely chemical 'solution' to schizophrenia

It has been said that 'most researchers continue to look for a purely biochemical solution, with the most recent candidates including glutamate, gamma-aminobutyric acid (GABA), and acetyl choline ...' While this is happening others researchers are said to be examining the, 'more productive path of linking biochemistry to the psychological and social domains' (Read, 2013, p. 66).

It is open to question whether 'most researchers' continue looking for a purely bio-chemical solution whatever a 'purely' biochemical 'solution' would look like (Read, 2013, p. 66). Researchers looking at the influence of neurochemicals are likely to focus on these in their work. But this does not preclude awareness of psychological and environmental influences, as Read (2013, p. 66) recognises.

For example, Howes and Kapur (2009) in developing version 3 of the dopamine hypothesis, 'the final common pathway' reviewed evidence in neurochemical imaging studies, genetic evidence, findings on environmental risk factors, research into the extended phenotype, and animal studies. Their hypothesis is that environmental stress and substance abuse interact with a genetic susceptibility, leading to dopamine dysregulation. Increases in striatal presynaptic dopamine concentration cause actual psychosis or proneness to it owing to aberrant salience to external stimuli.

As long ago as 2005, a 'social defeat' (SD) hypothesis was proposed taking SD as the negative experience of being excluded from the majority group (Selten and Cantor-Graae, 2005). It proposes that 'chronic and long-term' experience of SD may increase the risk of schizophrenia owing to sensitisation of the mesolimbic dopamine system and/or increased baseline activity of this system (Ibid.).

Later, Selten et al. (2013) updated literature relating to this hypothesis. They found that evidence for SD as a mechanism for increased risk of schizophrenia was strongest for migration and childhood trauma. Evidence was 'insufficient' for urban upbringing, low intelligence, and drug abuse. The researchers also looked at the evidence that long term exposure to SD leads to sensitisation of the mesolimbic system. Evidence relating to humans was 'insufficient' because there were too few studies, but the evidence regarding animals was 'strong.' It was argued that the SD hypothesis gives a 'parsimonious and plausible' explanation for several epidemiological findings not explained solely by 'genetic confounding' (Ibid.).

McCutcheon, Krystal and Howes (2020, p. 25) link social defeat factors and dopamine function. They note that 'measures of presynaptic dopamine function are raised in migrants, and those that have experienced childhood trauma, both of which are risk factors associated with schizophrenia' (Ibid., p. 25). None of this looks like researchers envisaging a purely chemical 'solution' to schizophrenia.

'Failed' neurochemical explanations undermine justifications for using antipsychotics

Critics may identify the dopamine theory as the 'cornerstone of biological psychiatry's claim that "schizophrenia" is an illness' and see it as the foundation of drug company marketing of antipsychotics' (Read, 2013, p. 66).

Commentators focusing on confirmation of the original dopamine theory having 'failed' can imply that schizophrenia is not an illness with neurochemical features. Consequently, the use of medication with a presumed action relating to dopamine dysregulation may not be justified. This would call into question the marketing of pharmaceutical companies basing their drug promotion solely on a claimed effect on the earlier proposed simple dopamine dysregulation.

However, the evolving dopamine hypothesis may support the use of medication which includes action on the dopamine system. Jauhar and colleagues (2017) state that their findings concerning the role of dopamine in schizophrenia (and other conditions) were consistent with a trans-diagnostic role for dopamine dysfunction in development of psychosis. They note that this suggests dopamine synthesis capacity as a potential novel drug target for schizophrenia (and bipolar disorder).

Conclusion

The 'original' dopamine hypothesis implicated excess dopamine in schizophrenia. However, dopamine metabolites were not universally elevated in the cerebrospinal fluid or serum of patients with schizophrenia, and autopsy studies of D2 receptors could not exclude the potential influence of previous antipsychotic treatment. Positive symptoms of schizophrenia appeared to be associated with subcortical release of dopamine which augments activation of the dopamine D2 receptor; and negative symptoms with reduced activation of the dopamine D1 receptor in the prefrontal cortex and decreased activity of the nucleus caudatus.

Version 2 pointed to brain areas involving excessive or depleted dopamine transmission. Overactivity of dopamine D2 receptor neurotransmission in subcortical and limbic brain regions contributes to a faulty emphasis being placed on some external stimuli manifesting itself in positive schizophrenia symptoms. Negative and cognitive symptoms were attributed to underactivity of dopamine D1 receptor neurotransmission in the prefrontal cortex. However, there was no direct evidence for low dopamine levels in the frontal cortex, limited direct evidence for elevated striatal dopamine function, and limited evidence of lower frontal levels of dopamine in schizophrenia.

Version 3 'the final common pathway' linked a wide range of risk factors to increased presynaptic striatal dopaminergic function. The hypothesis explains frontotemporal structural and functional abnormalities and cognitive impairments, and how these may converge neurochemically to cause psychosis through aberrant salience leading to a diagnosis of schizophrenia. It proposes that future drug research focuses on identifying and manipulating upstream factors converging on the dopaminergic funnel point. Difficulties arise concerning effects of previously taken antipsychotic medication, the potential confounding of results by stress and substance abuse, and possible bias involved in comparing healthy controls with inpatients with schizophrenia.

A stronger version 4 of the hypothesis could include more information on the role of dopamine, particularly how genetic and environmental factors combine to influence the common pathway, and point to better drugs directly influencing presynaptic dopaminergic function.

In criticisms of the evolving dopamine theory 'biological psychiatry' can become a limiting phrase conveying an over rigid perspective. Presenting 'too much dopamine' as being a still popular simplistic lead theory is out of date. It was proposed that the supposed continued 'failure' to confirm the original dopamine foremost hypothesis led to the investigation of other neurotransmitters, ignoring that evolution of earlier hypotheses led to consideration of other neurotransmitters.

Alternative neurochemical models and the interaction between dopamine, glutamate, GABA, acetylcholine, and serotonin are contributing to the development of understanding, without precluding any links between biochemistry and psychological and social domains. Implications for the use of medication including action on the dopamine system remain relevant. There may be a transdiagnostic role for dopamine dysfunction in the development of psychosis, suggesting that dopamine synthesis capacity may be a potential new drug target for schizophrenia and bipolar disorder.

Suggested further reading

Brisch, R., Saniotis, A., Wolf, R., Bielau, H., Bernstein, H.-G., Steiner, J., Bogerts, B., Braun, K., Jankowski, Z., Kumaratilake, J., Henneberg, M. and Gos, T. (2014) 'The role of dopamine in schizophrenia from a neurobiological and evolutionary perspective: Old fashioned, but still in vogue' *Frontiers in Psychiatry* (19 May 2014). https://www.ncbi.nlm.nih.gov/pmc/articles/PMC4032934/
Read, J. (2013) 'Biological psychiatry's lost cause: The 'schizophrenic' brain' in Read, J. and Dillon, J. (Eds.) (2nd Edition) *Models of Madness: Psychological, Social and Biological Approaches to Psychosis*. London and New York, Routledge (pp. 62–71).

References

Bhatia, A., Lenchner, J. R. and Saadabadi, A. (2021) 'Biochemistry, dopamine receptors' *The National Center for Biotechnology Information Resources* (Updated 22 July 2021). https://www.ncbi.nlm.nih.gov/books/NBK538242
Brisch, R., Saniotis, A., Wolf, R., Bielau, H., Bernstein, H.-G., Steiner, J., Bogerts, B., Braun, K., Jankowski, Z., Kumaratilake, J., Henneberg, M. and Gos, T. (2014) 'The role of dopamine in schizophrenia from a neurobiological and evolutionary perspective: Old fashioned, but still in vogue' *Frontiers in Psychiatry* (19 May 2014). https://www.ncbi.nlm.nih.gov/pmc/articles/PMC4032934/
Davis, K. L., Khan, R. S., Ko, G. and Davidson, M. (1991) 'Dopamine in schizophrenia: A review and reconceptualization' *American Journal of Psychiatry* 148, 1474–1486. https://pubmed.ncbi.nlm.nih.gov/1681750/
Hengartner, M. P. and Moncrieff, J. (2018) 'Inconclusive evidence in support of the dopamine hypothesis of psychosis: Why neurobiological research must

consider medication use, adjust for important confounders, choose stringent comparators, and use larger samples' *Frontiers in Psychiatry* (1 May 2018, Opinion article). https://www.frontiersin.org/articles/10.3389/fpsyt.2018.001 74/full

Howes, O. D. and Kapur, S. (2009) 'The dopamine hypothesis of schizophrenia: Version III—the final common pathway' *Schizophrenia Bulletin* 35, 3, 549–562. https://pubmed.ncbi.nlm.nih.gov/19325164/

Jauhar, S., Nour, M. M., Verones, M., Rogdaki, M., Bonoldi, I., Azis, M., Turkheimer, F., McGuire, P., Young, A. H. and Howes, O. D. (2017) 'A test of the transdiagnostic dopamine hypothesis of psychosis using positron emission tomographic imaging in bipolar affective disorder and schizophrenia' *JAMA Psychiatry* 74, 12, 1206–1213. https://www.semanticscholar.org/paper/A-Test-of-the-Transdiagnostic-Dopamine-Hypothesis-Jauhar-Nour/aadbe9adb12a2a7 131f1ce78f58025a5dc4abd2c

McCutcheon, R. A., Krystal, J. H. and Howes, O. D. (2020) 'Dopamine and glutamate in schizophrenia: Biology, symptoms and treatment' *World Psychiatry* 19, 15–33. https://pubmed.ncbi.nlm.nih.gov/31922684/

Read, J. (2013) 'Biological psychiatry's lost cause: The "schizophrenic" brain' in Read, J. and Dillon, J. (Eds.) (2nd Edition) *Models of Madness: Psychological, Social and Biological Approaches to Psychosis*. London and New York, Routledge (pp. 62–71).

Selten, J.-P. and Cantor-Graae, E. (2005) 'Social defeat: Risk factor in schizophrenia?' *British Journal of Psychiatry* 187, 101–102. https://pubmed.ncbi.nlm. nih.gov/16055818/

Selten, J.-P., van der Ven, E., Rutten, B. and Cantor-Graae, E. (2013) 'The Social Defeat Hypothesis of Schizophrenia: An Update' *Schizophrenia Bulletin* 39, 6, 1180–1186. https://pubmed.ncbi.nlm.nih.gov/24062592/

Stahl, S. M. (2018) 'Beyond the dopamine hypothesis: Dopamine, serotonin, and glutamate' *CNS Spectrums* 23, 187–191.

Yamada, S. (2022) *The Role of Serotonin in Schizophrenia*. Medscape. https:// www.medscape.org/viewarticle/423111

8
ANTIPSYCHOTICS

Introduction

After summarises aspects of orthodox and dissenting positions on the role of antipsychotic medication for schizophrenia, this chapter looks at the fortuitous development of chlorpromazine, the first antipsychotic drug. I describe different types of antipsychotics and their efficacy, looking at first- and second-generation drugs. For example, in a meta-analysis of multiple treatments, 15 antipsychotics were tested for efficacy and tolerability. Each were assigned a score based on the effect size of superiority to a placebo, the highest scores including clozapine and olanzapine. Adverse effects are discussed: sedation, weight gain, unwanted sexual effects, and movement disorders.

I examine the view that claims of certain pharmaceutical companies invite caution. A concern is sometimes expressed that the impartiality of some psychiatrists and groups to evaluate drug efficacy may be compromised by too close an association with big pharma. High financial benefits to drug companies and aggressive marketing create unease. Some pharmaceutical firms are accused of distorting their reporting of drug benefits. In the future, concerns may be alleviated by new codes of industry practice and other measures.

I discuss criticisms about administering antipsychotics. Dissenting voices may emphasise adverse effects rather than discuss strategies used by physicians for avoiding these, like differentiating between the risks associated with different antipsychotics. By contrast, orthodox practitioners may evaluate practicalities of choosing specific antipsychotics to reduce

DOI: 10.4324/9781003413554-8

the risk of adverse effects. For example, the least likely antipsychotics to cause sedation are aripiprazole, iloperidone, or paliperidone.

The chapter examines the argument that people with schizophrenia in developing countries do better with less access to antipsychotics. However, the picture is more complicated than at first appeared. Influential research suggests (at least) re-examining the prognosis of schizophrenia in low- and middle-income countries. I consider critics' views that no research confirms that antipsychotics 'fix' any known brain abnormality, or that they 'rebalance' brain chemistry, and that inflated claims about the ability of antipsychotics to 'cure' mental disorder are unsubstantiated. All this conforms to an orthodox view and is tilting at windmills. I provide an example of critics' use of inflated language regarding possible dampening effects of antipsychotics.

Orthodox and dissenting positions

An orthodox view tends to focus on the effectiveness of antipsychotic medication for example in comparison with a placebo. It is accepted that such medication does not 'cure' schizophrenia but addresses its symptoms. Side effects are recognised but so are efforts to select for patients anti-psychotics with a low risk of producing a particular side effect. It is noted that all second-generation antipsychotics and haloperidol were found to be 'more efficacious than placebo for overall symptoms of schizophrenia.' However, the effects were 'only of medium size' (Leucht et al., 2009, p. 164). Such drugs do not cure, rather, 'they *control* the symptoms of schizophrenia – as they do those of diabetes' (Torrey, 2019, p. 171, italics in original). When considering an antipsychotic, it is accepted that side effects should be a 'primary consideration' (Torrey, 2019, p. 177). Also, side effects are balanced against, 'the severity of the basic disease' (Moller and Riedel, 2009, p. 231).

A dissenting position tends to emphasise that antipsychotics do not cure schizophrenia or 'fix' a brain abnormality, claims which orthodox prac-titioners do not make. It may be accepted that antipsychotics 'help certain people some of the time.' However, claims that they can cure mental disorder are 'unsubstantiated' (Davies, 2014, p. 287). Also, research does not show that antipsychotics 'fix any known brain abnormality,' or optimally 'rebalance brain chemistry' (Ibid., p. 288). Dissenters depict antipsychotics as 'diminishing' functions that are 'integral to our mental activity.' Davies (2014, pp. 288–289) quoting a patient says that an individual must decide whether 'paying with one's soul is an acceptable price' for having symptoms mitigated.

Antipsychotics: discovery, types and effectiveness, and action

The fortuitous development of chlorpromazine the first antipsychotic drug

Chlorpromazine, which became the first antipsychotic, did not start out as such. Synthesised in 1951 in the Rhône-Poulenc pharmaceutical company laboratories, it was released for clinical investigation in May 1952 as a possible potentiator of general anaesthesia. Chlorpromazine's potential use in psychiatry was first recognised by French army surgeon Henri Laborit. During his research with artificial hibernation to prevent surgical shock, he found that the drug, administered intravenously, produced disinterest without loss of consciousness (Ban, 2007, p. 495).

Knowing that in France lowering a patient's temperature with cold water was a remedy to control agitation and believing (incorrectly) that the drug action involved a cooling effect, Laborit persuaded colleagues of the neuro-psychiatric service of the Paris military hospital to try chlorpromazine in treating one of their patients. In this way, a 24-year-old 'manic' psychiatric patient became the first to receive the drug. In November 1952, chlorpromazine became available on prescription in France, under the proprietary name of Largactil (meaning 'large action'). Its effectiveness transformed the provision in so-called 'disturbed wards,' while its commercial success encouraged the development of other psychotropic drugs (Ban, 2007, pp. 495–496).

Types of antipsychotics and their efficacy

A distinction is made between first-generation antipsychotics (FGAs) and second-generation antipsychotics (SGAs). First-generation ('typical') antipsychotics were produced prior to 1990, while second-generation ('atypical') ones were made subsequently. Antipsychotics are available as pills to be taken orally, or in long-acting injectable form.

In a meta-analysis of multiple treatments, 15 antipsychotics were tested for efficacy and tolerability in 212 trials. Each drug was assigned a score based on the effect size of being better than a placebo (Leucht et al., 2013). The first few highest effect scores are shown below – generic name first, trade name following in round brackets, effectiveness score in square brackets. All are second-generation drugs except haloperidol.

clozapine (Clozaril)	[88]
olanzapine (Zyprexa)	[59]
risperidone (Risperdal)	[56]
paliperidone (Invega)	[50]
haloperidol (Haldol)	[45]

Antipsychotics help to control some of the symptoms of schizophrenia. They do not 'cure' or 'fix' the condition, nor is there any claim that they do so. If taken as prescribed, antipsychotics can reduce the chance of relapse. For example, a review of 65 studies indicated that at the end of one year, that only 27% of people with schizophrenia taking antipsychotics had relapsed, while a much larger 64% of people with schizophrenia not taking antipsychotics had relapsed (Leucht et al., 2012).

A broad view of the potential effectiveness of and variations in antipsychotics is provided by Mind, a UK mental health charity. After describing psychotic symptoms, the organisation states that, 'antipsychotics might not get rid of these symptoms completely' but may prevent the user, 'feeling so bothered by them.' This can help users 'feel more stable' so that they can get on with life as they wish. Antipsychotics, it is noted, can reduce the risk of relapse. Some types of antipsychotic work better than others for specific symptoms. Also, 'you may find that antipsychotics aren't right for you' (Mind, 2022).

The action of antipsychotics

Antipsychotics target brain neurotransmitter receptors, particularly dopamine (DA). Produced in the brain's substantia nigra and ventral tegmental regions, dopamine has different functions in mesolimbic, mesocortical, nigrostriatal, and tuberoinfundibular pathways. These neuronal connections allow dopamine to pass on information involving cognition, executive thinking, voluntary motor movements, and feelings of pleasure and reward. Dopamine receptors are expressed in the central nervous system (hippocampal dentate gyrus, and subventricular zone) and in the periphery, including the kidney. Five types of dopamine receptors each have various functions:

D1: memory, attention, impulse control, regulation of renal function, locomotion
D2: locomotion, attention, sleep, memory, learning
D3: cognition, impulse control, attention, sleep
D4: cognition, impulse control, attention, sleep
D5: decision making, cognition, attention, renin secretion (Bhatia, Lenchner and Saadabadi, 2021).

Some antipsychotics also implicate other receptors including serotonin, which is involved in modulating mood, cognition, reward, memory, and learning.

The action of first-generation antipsychotics

First-generation antipsychotics like chlorpromazine were considered to act by blocking D2 receptors in the mesolimbic dopamine pathway so reducing the positive symptoms of schizophrenia. However, by also inhibiting D2 receptors in other dopamine pathways, they could cause side effects. For example, inhibiting D2 receptors in the mesocortical dopamine pathway can worsen negative symptoms.

Receptors in the nigrostriatal DA pathway which are involved in the extrapyramidal system can, when inhibited, result in extrapyramidal symptoms. These include acute dystonic reactions involving involuntary muscle contractions of the face, neck, trunk, pelvis, and limbs. Blocking D2 receptors in the tuberoinfundibular DA pathway can lead to hyperprolactinaemia. This involves raised levels of blood prolactin which can create problems including in women breast pain, and menstrual irregularities, and in men, sexual dysfunction. Where first-generation antipsychotics also blocked other neurotransmission systems, this too could lead to adverse effects (Lee and Chang, 2009, p. 219).

The action of second-generation antipsychotics

Pharmaceutically, second-generation antipsychotics can be defined as serotonin dopamine antagonists, as D2 antagonists with rapid association, and as D2 partial antagonists. Importantly for second-generation antipsychotics, the secretion of dopamine from dopaminergic neurons is inhibited by serotonin binding to serotonin 2A (5HT2A) receptors. Most second-generation antipsychotics act by antagonising both the DA receptor and the 5HT2A receptor. To illustrate this action, we can consider serotonin dopamine antagonists in three pathways:

- nigrostriatal
- mesocortical, and
- tuberoinfundibular.

In the nigrostriatal pathway, serotonin dopamine antagonists block D2 receptors and 5HT2A receptors aiding the release of dopamine. Following this, in the synapse, dopamine (released through the serotonin receptor being blocked) can compete with the serotonin dopamine antagonists for the D2 receptor. This causes a reverse of the D2 antagonism of serotonin dopamine antagonists. These activities of serotonin dopamine antagonists attenuate extrapyramidal symptoms which were a side effect of first-generation antipsychotics, blocking D2 in the nigrostriatal pathway (Lee and Chang, 2009, p. 220 and figure 18.2).

In the mesocortical dopamine pathway of people with schizophrenia, where relatively low levels of dopamine and higher levels of serotonin may be found, serotonin dopamine antagonists dominantly inhibit the serotonin receptor. This leads to release of dopamine and subsequently improvement in negative and cognitive symptoms (Ibid.).

Turning to the tuberoinfundibular pathway, pituitary lactotroph cells release prolactin which is inhibited by dopamine but induced by serotonin. While first-generation antipsychotics could induce prolactin secretion though blockading D2 causing hyperprolactinemia, it appears that serotonin dopamine antagonists can reduce prolactin secretion though its 5HT2A antagonism so alleviating hyperprolactinemia (Ibid.).

Broadly, the action of second-generation antipsychotics can mitigate some side effects associated with first-generation antipsychotics. Side effects however remain an important consideration in administering antipsychotics as we now discuss.

Side effects of antipsychotics

Antipsychotics differ in the adverse effects that they can produce, making these a major consideration in indicating which antipsychotics might be prescribed. Potential side effects include:

- weight gain
- sedation
- movement disorders, and
- sexual side effects.

Weight gain

A major side effect of antipsychotics is weight gain. Often accompanied by increase in blood sugar and in blood lipids, it is a risk factor for heart attacks and strokes. Should blood sugar increase to very high levels, it results in potentially fatal ketoacidosis as the body produces high levels of blood acids (ketones). Increases in weight and in blood sugar levels occur more commonly in people taking clozapine (Clozaril) and olanzapine (Zyprexa). In good practice, the treating psychiatrist takes a baseline weight of a patient starting antipsychotics. When administering clozapine (Clozaril) and olanzapine (Zyprexa) good practice indicates also taking a baseline blood sugar and haemoglobin. Advice from a dietician and increased exercise also contribute to weight control, especially in the first few months of taking antipsychotics (Torrey, 2019, p. 177).

Sedation

Sedation can hinder daily living, including work, and for some people can give a feeling of being diminished. Severest when starting the antipsychotic, sedation tends to become less so later. Effects can be reduced if the medication is taken at bedtime. Several antipsychotics for example aripiprazole (Abilify) are identified as least likely to produce sedation.

Movement disorders

Various unpleasant movement disorders (extrapyramidal symptoms) may occur as side effects of antipsychotics. These include acute dystonic reactions involving sustained or intermittent involuntary muscle contractions of the face, neck, trunk, pelvis, and limbs. This is quickly reversible by anticholinergic drugs. Consequently, these drugs are sometimes given preventively with antipsychotics that are more likely to cause dystonic reactions. Another movement disorder that may occur is akathisia, a compelling urge to move about leading to pacing and restlessness.

Most serious of movement disorders that may occur is tardive dyskinesia. It typically involves irregular movements of the tongue, lips, jaw, and face, and, in some instances, the peri-orbital areas (between the upper and mid face). Sometimes the person develops irregular trunk and limb movements. Characteristically, the movements are jerking, writhing, and twitching. The prefix 'tardive' (late onset) conveys that the condition is more common in people who have received antipsychotics for a prolonged time. Also, tardive dyskinesia tends to appear in older people after a comparatively short period of antipsychotic treatment (Ricciardi et al., 2019, p. 389).

Preventing or mitigating symptoms of tardive dyskinesia involves following best practice for prescribing antipsychotic medication. This includes limiting the prescription for specific indications, using the minimum effective dose, and minimising the duration of therapy. In managing tardive dyskinesia, antipsychotic medication is withdrawn if practicable, although for many patients with serious mental disorder, this is not feasible owing to relapse. Switching from a first-generation to a second-generation antipsychotic with a lower dopamine D2 affinity, like clozapine, may reduce symptoms (Ricciardi et al., 2019, p. 389).

Sexual side effects

Some antipsychotics may produce sexual side effects. By increasing the hormone prolactin, they can cause slight breast enlargement, breast discharges, irregularities in menstruation, and sexual dysfunction. Long-term elevation of prolactin may also cause osteoporosis, weakening the bones and making them fragile. Several antipsychotics for example quetiapine (Seroquel) are identified as having a lower risk than others of producing prolactin.

Some research and claims associated with pharmaceutical companies invite caution

Concerns about medication use include worries about the involvement of large pharmaceutical companies. Concern about some aspects of the involvement of pharmaceutical companies is expressed not only by some critics, but also by some orthodox practitioners.

Critics maintain that the impartiality of some psychiatrists and groups to evaluate the efficacy of certain drugs may be impaired by too close an association with pharmaceutical companies. High financial benefits to drug companies and aggressive marketing also create worries. Accusations of pharmaceutical firms distorting the reporting of drug benefits damage the reputations of some companies.

Typical of such views are comments by (Davies, 2014). Who maintains that drug firms are, 'notoriously secretive.' They have a record of not being open about how drugs are developed and marketed and of, 'concealing negative trials that show their drugs in a bad light' (Ibid., p. 88). He describes AstraZeneca's discovery in early 2000 that its most recent research into Seroquel indicated the drug to be 'far less effective' than its competitor Haldol (Ibid., p. 148).

In response, the company adopted 'cherry picking' by which only some of the data from a clinical trial are published.

Davies (2014) points out that after a year taking Seroquel, patients experienced 'more relapses' and lower ratings on symptom scales than those on Haldol. They also gained weight increasing risk of diabetes. Rather than 'admitting' this, the company focused on, 'one shred of positive data about the drug faring slightly better on some measures of cognitive functioning' (Ibid., pp. 150–151). Davies (2014) observes, by 2010 many people taking Seroquel were experiencing, 'awful side effects' and that around 17,500 claimed that the firm 'had lied about the risks of the drug.' In 2010, AstraZeneca paid £125 million to settle 'a class action out of court for defrauding the public' (Ibid., p. 152).

Broader criticism is presented by Goldacre (2012) in *Bad Pharma: How Drug Companies Mislead Doctors and Harm Patients*. He expresses concern about the process of getting pharmaceuticals licensed for clinical use, then maximising their use by treating physicians and patients. This has too often compromised study design and the open sharing of data about study results. National drug regulatory organisations have not always ensured that studies have focused on the right groups of patients, that cost, and effectiveness are fully considered, and that value is added to existing treatments.

Such criticism of some pharmaceutical companies is shared by some orthodox practitioners and dissenters, although perhaps dissenters are more sceptical about suggestions to rectify matters. Among proposals to improve matters are the development of new codes of industry practice, ensuring open-access disclosure by prescribers and clinical trialists who get industry funding, and a requirement of open access to full clinical trial data.

Dissenting views of antipsychotics and some weaknesses

Dissenting views tend to be critical of the use of antipsychotics, although some of these criticisms have their own weaknesses. Critics may:

- emphasise adverse effects of antipsychotics rather how to reduce or avoid these
- place undue weight on claims that those with schizophrenia in developing countries do better with less access to antipsychotics
- criticise supposed orthodox views that are not in fact held ('tilting at windmills')
- use overstated language.

Emphasising adverse effects of antipsychotics rather how to reduce or avoid them

Antipsychotics undoubtedly can cause unpleasant side effects. This is common ground between orthodox practitioners and critics. However, orthodox and dissenting advocates may differ in the attention paid to choices available among different antipsychotics, and practical steps to mitigate adverse effects.

For example, in their chapter on, 'Antipsychotic drugs' Hutton et al. (2013) discuss adverse effects. Under 'first-generation antipsychotics' the authors cover tardive dyskinesia, and neuroleptic malignant syndrome. In considering 'second-generation antipsychotics' they cite cardiovascular effects and blood problems, extrapyramidal effects, metabolic effects (like weight gain and sexual dysfunction), reductions in brain volume, and mortality (Ibid., pp. 110–116). Looking at weight gain, the chapter mentions the various levels of risk of different drugs. The authors note the 'high variability' in metabolic effects caused by different antipsychotics and that the highest risk is associated with olanzapine, clozapine, and quetiapine.

They cite a Clinical Antipsychotic Trials of Intervention Effectiveness (CATIE) study sponsored by the US National Institute of Mental Health. Risks of weight gain were identified for a range of antipsychotics. Weight gain more than 7% after 18 months occurred among 30% of people treated with olanzapine and 7% with ziprasidone. Hutton et al. (2013) observe, 'This situation is concerning because metabolic syndrome doubles the 10-year risk of coronary heart disease' (Ibid., p. 114). While risks were mentioned ranging from 30% to 7% there was no indication of implications for patient and clinician choosing an antipsychotic with lowest risk. What is mentioned instead is that the risks are 'concerning' because of the effect of metabolic syndrome on the risk of coronary heart disease.

By contrast, Torrey (2019) discusses side effects of antipsychotics but also practicalities of choosing specific antipsychotics to reduce risk of adverse effects. He observes, 'It is now widely accepted that the primary consideration in selecting antipsychotics should be side effects' (Ibid., p. 177).

Regarding the movement disorders grouped as extra pyramidal symptom (EPS), it is noted that clozapine (Clozaril), quetiapine (Seroquel), olanzapine (Zyprexa), and thioridazine (Melanil) are 'the least likely to cause EPS' (Ibid., p. 178).

Some antipsychotics cause sexual side effects such as breast discharge and sexual dysfunction by increasing the hormone prolactin. However, several are 'least likely to increase prolactin' including aripiprazole (Abilify) and quetiapine (Seroquel). Furthermore, sedation problems can be mitigated by taking the drug at bedtime (Torrey, 2019, p. 180).

Weight gain as a side effect is often accompanied by increased blood sugar and increased lipids which is a risk factor in heart attacks and strokes. Among the least likely to cause such problems are haloperidol (Haldol) and fluphenazine (Prolixin) (Torrey, 2019, p. 171). Also, it is 'good practice' for the treating psychiatrist to get a baseline weight on any patient starting antipsychotics. For those taking clozapine (Clozaril) or olanzapine (Zyprexa), it is good practice to take a baseline of blood sugar and haemoglobin (Ibid., p. 177). Patients taking drugs that can cause weight gain should be referred to a dietician for dietary advice and should increase their exercise (Ibid.).

Claims that those with schizophrenia in developing countries do better with less access to antipsychotics – overlooking contrary evidence

It is sometimes suggested in press coverage (e.g., Whitaker, 2010) that in third-world countries schizophrenia has a better outcome than in first-word countries, including when the disorder is not treated with antipsychotics. However, it emerges that the picture is more complicated than such dichotomising suggests.

Cohen et al. (2008) reconsider whether progress for schizophrenia is better in the developing world, a view that has, 'become an axiom in international psychiatry.' Maintaining such a position would be 'unfortunate given increasing evidence, which presents a far more complex picture.' Their review considered people with schizophrenia living in low- and middle-income countries. It examined 'clinical outcomes and patterns of course, disability and social outcomes, and mortality and suicide.' Also considered was evidence concerning family roles, effects of gender, and the interpretation of evidence about people with schizophrenia who 'have not received biomedical treatment' (Ibid., p. 229). It would be sensible, the researchers conclude, in comparing low- and middle-income countries, to discard 'presumed wisdom' and revisit the seeming prognosis of schizophrenia (Ibid., Conclusions).

Cohen and colleagues (2008) representation of data which largely informed their observations is challenged. Indicating the complexity of some of the findings, Jablensky and Sartorius (2008) accept that patient outcome in developing countries was 'not uniformly better' compared with that of developed countries. High rates of 'complete clinical remission' in developing countries were significantly more common than in developed countries. However, when compared with patients in developed counties, patients in developing ones had 'significantly longer periods of unimpaired functioning in the community.' This was so despite only 16% being on continuous antipsychotics while in developed countries, the figure was 61% (Ibid.).

Further evidence suggests caution in claiming that in third-world countries schizophrenia has a better outcome than in first-word countries, including when not treated with antipsychotics. Sullivan, Allen and Nero (2007) studying schizophrenia in Palau a Republic in the western Pacific note that the republic has 'one of the highest rates of schizophrenia in the world.' Their results are used to challenges a view arising from earlier cross-cultural research that 'the expression of schizophrenia in necessarily more benign in "developing" countries' (Ibid., p. 189).

Alem and colleagues (2009) examined the clinical course and outcome of schizophrenia in rural Ethiopia. The researchers acknowledge that outcome in that setting seems better than in developed countries. However, they note that only a low proportion of participants were in complete remission. This indicates that outcome of schizophrenia in developing countries may be 'heterogeneous rather than uniformly favourable.' The researchers suggest outcomes in rural Ethiopia may be improved by better access to treatment (Ibid., p. 654). They observe that the 'overall pattern' of outcome of schizophrenia in rural Ethiopia is similar to that found in developing countries. Nevertheless, the community-based study showed a 'clear tendency toward a poorer outcome.' Noting that antipsychotics crucially modify outcomes of 'severe mental disorders,' the researchers state that ensuring 'adequate treatment and enhancement of adherence should receive priority' (Ibid.).

Citing inflated claims for antibiotics that are not held tilting at windmills

There is a certain amount of rhetoric in dissenting language in relation to antipsychotics.

Davies (2014) as shown already provides examples. It is not part of the orthodox position to claim that antibiotics cure ('fix') schizophrenia, but rather that the drugs reduce certain of the symptoms. Neither is it held that antipsychotics rebalance brain chemicals to an optimum level – developments in the dopamine hypotheses for example have evolved into more precise understandings (see Chapter 7).

So, for Davies to say that '... there is no research confirming that antipsychotics fix any known brain abnormality, or that they 'rebalance' brain chemistry to some optimum level' is irrelevant to current debates (Davies, 2014, p. 288). Similarly, it is stated with regard to antipsychotics that 'inflated claims about their ability to "cure" mental disorder are unsubstantiated' (Ibid., p. 287). Here not only is it obvious that antipsychotics do not offer a cure, but it is surely also evident that inflated claims about anything are (by definition) unsubstantiated.

Faustian descriptions of sedation – overstated language

Davies (2014) accepts that using antipsychotics leads to 'a reduction in the intensity of psychotic symptoms.' Antipsychotics also, as he points out, have a sedating effect. He expresses this as that they, 'diminish other physical, emotional functions integral to all our mental activity.'

But picking up a quote from a patient who disliked the effect of antipsychotics, Davies observes, 'It is of course up to the individual patient to decide whether **paying with one's soul** is an acceptable price to pay for the mitigation of their symptoms' (Ibid., p. 288–289, bold added). How such Faustian allusions of paying with one's soul carries forward debate is unclear. It may be good rhetoric but makes a weak argument as overstatement.

Conclusion

The discovery of chlorpromazine, which became the first antipsychotic drug, was serendipitous. It was originally thought (incorrectly) to have a cooling action which might calm people with schizophrenia. Following chlorpromazine first-generation antipsychotics were developed and later, second-generation drugs. Different antipsychotics differ in efficacy. In a meta-analysis of multiple treatments, antipsychotics tested for efficacy and tolerability were each assigned a score based on the effect size of being better than a placebo. Among the highest effect scores were clozapine, olanzapine, risperidone, paliperidone, and haloperidol. Antipsychotics can cause various adverse side effects, namely sedation, weight gain, unwanted sexual effects, and movement disorders.

Some clinicians and others, whether orthodox or dissenting, question the impartiality of certain psychiatrists and groups. The issue is whether they can impartially evaluate the efficacy of particular drugs because of a too close an association with pharmaceutical companies. Among concerns are high financial benefits to drug companies, aggressive marketing, and accusations of companies distorting the reporting of drug benefits. Possible strategies to improve matters are new codes of industry practice, ensuring open-access disclosure by prescribers and clinical trialists who get industry funding, and a requirement of open access to full clinical trial data.

Critics may emphasise adverse effects of antipsychotics rather than discuss how clinicians can avoiding or mitigate such effects, for example by differentiating between the risks associated with different antipsychotics and by using other measures. By contrast, orthodox practitioners may fully consider practicalities of choosing specific antipsychotics to reduce the risk of adverse effects.

For example, weight gain as a side effect is often accompanied by increased blood sugar and increased lipids which is a risk factor in heart attacks and strokes. Varied risk of different drugs may be recognised affecting different percentages of people ranging from 30% (olanzapine) to 7% (ziprasidone). Other steps are getting a baseline weight on any patient starting antipsychotics, and a baseline of blood sugar and haemoglobin for those taking clozapine or olanzapine. Patients can be referred to a dietician for dietary advice and should increase their exercise.

The view held by some critics that people with schizophrenia in developing countries do better with less access to antipsychotics has been challenged. Influential research has suggested re-examining the question of the prognosis of schizophrenia in low- and middle-income countries.

Some critics tilt at windmills in stating that no research confirms that antipsychotics 'fix' any known brain abnormality, or that they 'rebalance' brain chemistry, and that inflated claims about the ability of antipsychotics to 'cure' mental disorder are unsubstantiated. Inflated language may be used, apocalyptically describing possible dampening effects of antipsychotics.

Suggested further reading

Davies, J. (2014) *Cracked: Why Psychiatry Is Doing More Harm than Good.* London, Icon Books.
Torrey, E. F. (2019) (7th Edition) *Surviving Schizophrenia: A Family Manual.* New York and London, Harper Perennial.

References

Alem, A., Kebede, D., Fekadu, A., Shibre, T., Fekadu, D., Beyero, T., Medhin, G., Negash, A. and Kullgren, G. (2009) 'Clinical course and outcome of schizophrenia in a predominantly treatment-naïve cohort in rural Ethiopia' *Schizophrenia Bulletin* 35, 646–654. https://www.ncbi.nlm.nih.gov/pmc/articles/PMC2669573/
Ban, T. A. (2007) 'Fifty years of chlorpromazine: A historical perspective' *Neuropsychiatric Disease and Treatment* 3, 4, 495–500. https://pubmed.ncbi.nlm.nih.gov/19300578/
Cohen, A., Patel, V., Thara, R. and Gureje, O. (2008) 'Questioning an axiom: Better prognosis for schizophrenia in the developing world?' *Schizophrenia Bulletin* 34, 229–244. https://www.ncbi.nlm.nih.gov/pmc/articles/PMC2632419/
Davies, J. (2014) *Cracked: Why Psychiatry Is Doing More Harm than Good.* London, Icon Books.
Goldacre, B. (2012) *Bad Pharma: How Drug Companies Mislead Doctors and Harm Patients.* London, Fourth Estate.
Hutton, P., Weinmann, S., Bola, J. and Read, J. (2013) 'Antipsychotic drugs' in Read, J. and Dillon, J. (Eds.) (2nd Edition) *Models of Madness: Psychological, Social and Biological Approaches to Psychosis.* London and New York, Routledge.
Jablensky, A. and Sartorius, N. (2008) 'What did the WHO studies really find?' *Schizophrenia Bulletin* 34, 2, 253–255. https://www.semanticscholar.org/paper/What-Did-the-WHO-Studies-Really-Find-Jablensky-Sartorius/c375847ae99e0b55 19bc0a35ba4b2a6ccba3ca38
Lee, M.-S. and Chang, H. S. (2009) 'Pharmacological profile and pharmacogenetic approaches of antipsychotics' in Kasper, S. and Papadimitriou, G. N. (Eds.) (2nd Edition) *Schizophrenia: Biopsychosocial Approaches and Current Challenges* (Medical Psychiatry Series). New York and London, Informa Healthcare (pp. 218–230).
Leucht, S., Corves, C., Kissling, W. and Davies, J. M. (2009) 'An update of meta-analyses on second generation antipsychotic drugs for schizophrenia' in Kasper, S. and Papadimitriou, G. N. (Eds.) (2nd Edition) *Schizophrenia: Biopsychosocial*

Approaches and Current Challenges (Medical Psychiatry Series). New York and London, Informa Healthcare (pp. 164–173).

Leucht, S., Tardy, M., Komossa, K., Heres, S., Kissling, W., Salanti, G. and Davis, J. M. (2012) 'Antipsychotic drugs versus placebo for relapse prevention in schizophrenia: A systematic review and meta-analysis' *Lancet* 379, 2063–2071 https://www.thelancet.com/pdfs/journals/lancet/PIIS0140-6736(12)60239-6.pdf

Leucht, S., Cipriani, A., Spineli, L., Mavridis, D., Orey, D., Richter, F., Samara, M., Barbui, C., Engel, R. R., Geddes, J. R., Kissling, W., Stapf, M. P., Lässig, B., Salanti, G. and Davis, J. M. (2013) 'Comparative efficacy and tolerability of 15 antipsychotic drugs in schizophrenia: A multiple-treatments meta-analysis' *Lancet* 382, 951–962. https://www.thelancet.com/journals/lancet/article/PIIS0140-6736(13)60733-3/fulltext

Mind (2022) 'Antipsychotics' Mind. https://www.mind.org.uk/information-support/drugs-and-treatments/antipsychotics/about-antipsychotics/

Moller, H.-J. and Riedel, M. (2009) 'Side-effect burden of antipsychotic medication' in Kasper, S. and Papadimitriou, G. N. (Eds.) (2009) (2nd Edition) *Schizophrenia: Biopsychosocial Approaches and Current Challenges* (Medical Psychiatry Series). New York and London, Informa Healthcare (pp. 231–259).

Rang, H. (2012) Review of *Bad Pharma: How Drug Companies Mislead Doctors and Harm Patients British Journal of Clinical Pharmacology.* https://www.ncbi.nlm.nih.gov/pmc/articles/PMC3635613/

Ricciardi, L., Pringsheim, T., Barnes, T. R. E., Martino, D., Gardner, D. Remington, G., Addington, D., Morgante, F., Poole, N., Carson, A. and Edwards, M. (2019) 'Treatment recommendations for Tardive Dyskinesia' *The Canadian Journal of Psychiatry* 64, 6, 388–399. https://journals.sagepub.com/doi/full/10.1177/0706743719828968

Sullivan, R. J., Allen, J. S. and Nero, K. L. (2007) 'Schizophrenia in Palau: A biocultural analysis' *Current Anthropology* 48, 189–213. https://www.semanticscholar.org/paper/Schizophrenia-in-Palau-Sullivan-Allen/223ecf7cd81d759e06ff4fddcdcd5322a9e09584

Torrey, E. F. (2019) (7th edition) *Surviving Schizophrenia: A Family Manual.* New York and London, Harper Perennial.

Whitaker, R. (2010) *Anatomy of an Epidemic: Magic Bullets, Psychiatric Drugs, and the Astonishing Rise of Mental Illness in America.* New York, Crown.

9

THE CONTINUING ROLE OF ELECTROCONVULSIVE THERAPY (ECT)

Introduction

This chapter illustrates polarised positive and negative personal accounts of ECT from decades ago, noting reports of similar extremes of experience on the internet today. I then turn to the broader, more consistently positive, current picture of patient perspectives from surveys and elsewhere. Outlining the modern procedures for administering ECT, I include its brief duration, and options for placing head electrodes. The chapter examines how ECT might work, including the theory that seizure activity in the limbic system induces neurotrophic effects (relating to the growth of nervous tissue).

Conditions treated with ECT are mentioned including its occasional use with schizophrenia, for example for catatonia, when other treatments have proved ineffective, and the condition is life threatening. Some recent studies are cited showing the positive effects of ECT, including open studies and chart reviews of more than 850 patients. They indicate that a combination ECT and antipsychotics is more effective than either antipsychotics or ECT alone.

Turning to criticisms of ECT efficacy, the chapter looks at the negative, emotive colouring of descriptions of pioneer work on ECT. Next, I suggest that critics may overlook limitations of some earlier studies that suggested poor ECT efficacy, especially where they preceded improvements in procedures and monitoring of ECT reflected in modern guidance. The chapter looks at critics' potentially misleading reference to dates of research, masking that old studies are cited.

DOI: 10.4324/9781003413554-9

Risks relating to ECT are discussed. Regarding memory loss, current UK guidance recognises that ECT may cause memory impairment for past and current events. However, memory impairment being a feature of many mental health problems it may sometimes be difficult to attribute. Cognitive impairment may occur both immediately after administration of ECT and following a course of therapy, which may distress those affected. Some people find their memory loss extremely damaging, negating for them any benefit from ECT.

I point out that current evaluations conclude that there is no evidence suggesting that mortality from ECT is greater than that of minor procedures using general anaesthetics. The chapter notes that, in discussing ECT and brain damage, critics tend to have different interpretations of research than orthodox commentators. They may use emotive language adding nothing to debate. Also considered is that current UK guidance found that six reviewed studies using brain-scanning techniques provided no evidence that ECT causes brain damage.

Orthodox and dissenting positions

Orthodox practitioners generally hold a more positive view of the efficacy and suitability of ECT than dissenters, while recognising that the treatment may be appropriate only in limited circumstances. They are careful to refer to contemporary research. For example, it is stated that ECT can be a 'very useful strategy' especially for people with 'affective or pharmacological treatment resistant symptoms.' Also, strong improvements have been reported in life-threatening conditions like malignant catatonia which indicate the importance of ECT as a possible treatment (Petrides and Braga, 2009, pp. 295–296). Indeed, ECT remains a 'valuable, irreplaceable treatment option' (Kaliora, Zervas and Papadimitriou, 2018, pp. 291–302). Orthodox practitioners consider that there is 'no evidence that ECT causes damage to the brain' (Torrey, 2019, p. 197). Information about ECT should be contemporary because old evidence can 'distort people's perspectives.' Importantly, public perceptions can affect attitudes to patients getting ECT and influence stigma and discrimination sometimes linked with receiving it. The views of prospective and actual patients receiving ECT are important in that they can influence the 'choice of treatment, consent to treatment, and self-stigma' (Griffiths and O'Niell-Kerr, 2019).

Dissenters tend to reject ECT as a treatment option, believing that it is not effective and causes brain damage. It is said that many psychiatrists are convinced of the efficacy of ECT, their claims are offset by 'reams of research' that indicate that the treatment has ill effects, poor rates of remission, and causes 'neurological damage' (Davies, 2014, p. 211).

Research has been carried out comparing the improvement rates of real and fake ECT. Six months later, assessment was done using the Hamilton Scale (a rating scale for depression). This showed a two-point difference in favour of the fake treatment. This was taken to suggest that any positive changes were 'largely placebo effects' (Davies, 2014, pp. 211–212, citing Bracken et al., 2012). It is claimed that responsible for the 'electro-shocking' of numerous people has been 'simplistic' genetic and biological theories (Read, Mosher and Bentall, 2013, p. 3).

Patient perspectives of ECT

Sasha, 30, a married schoolteacher, experienced severe depression. After being treated with different medications, in the year 2000, doctors suggested ECT as seemingly the only remaining option. Sasha says that she could not 'get through 5 minutes of the day without thinking about dying.' She noticed the difference after her first ECT treatment.

After her scheduled six sessions, she felt she was 'back to the same person I used to be.' Sasha went back to work and performed fine. She says of ECT, 'I can truly say that it saved my life' (Tracy, 2022a).

Juli Lawrence had ECT for depression in 1994 and was re-diagnosed as having bipolar disorder during the ECT treatments. Following her negative experience, a year later, she created a website SHOCKED!ECT. Juli says that, according to her mother, the ECT 'lifted me from a depression into a brief silliness.' This was the 'euphoric high' that can be experienced following ECT. However, this was soon succeeded by 'an even worse depression than before.' Juli says that the treatment left her with 'severe memory loss, and I believe some cognitive damage' (Tracy, 2022b).

These polarised, vivid accounts of personal experiences of ECT refer to decades ago, when procedures differed from contemporary ones. However, recent personal accounts on the internet tend to be similarly polarised, varying from horror stories to promotional material for health services. This suggests looking beyond individual accounts to a broader, contemporary picture of patient perspectives of ECT. Indeed, researchers recognise that the views of people who might gain benefit from ECT and current ECT patients are important 'because they can determine choice of treatment, consent to treatment, and self-stigma' (Griffiths and O'Niell-Kerr, 2019).

Surveys of patients having had ECT treatment reveal positive attitudes to effectiveness (Rush, McCarron and Lucey, 2007; Rayner et al., 2009). One study reported that fewer that a fifth of respondents rated ECT as slightly or much worse than a dentist visit. Some 97% did not report the experience to be very stressful (Benbow and Crentsil, 2004). Support for further sessions of ECT were high (Rayner et al., 2009). However, the majority of patients consider that relief of depressive symptoms is transient, and repeated treatments are required (Smith et al., 2009).

Improvements have been made in pre-treatment information, allaying fears, reducing feelings of coercion, and involving patients in treatment choice. An old 1976 review indicated that only 21% of patients reported that they were given adequate information prior to treatment (Freeman and Kendall, 1980). By contrast, a 2004 study found that around 80% of patients found the treatment had been fairly well or very well explained (Benbow and Crentsil, 2004). In a 2007 study, 85% stated that written information about the treatment was helpful (Rush, McCarron and Lucey, 2007).

Initiatives by the ECT accreditation service of the Royal College of Psychiatrists (ECTAS) and the Scottish ECT accreditation network have improved the quality of information given to patients prior to their treatment. The ECTAS report (2013–2015) noted 'significant improvements in practice since the inception of the scheme.' A total of 202 patient questionnaires were returned to ECTAS on the effectiveness of ECT. Some 77% of respondents said, 'yes' to the question 'did ECT help you?'; while only 12% said 'no.' The rest responded, 'don't know/can't remember' (Royal College of Psychiatrists, 2016).

Perhaps relatedly, newspapers have begun to cover modern ECT practices and contemporary personal experiences of ECT, describing positive aspects both from carer and patient perspectives (Talon, 2012; Davis, 2017; Smith, 2018).

ECT and its application

Modern ECT procedures and their brief duration

ECT involves electrically inducing a generalised seizure without muscular convulsions to manage certain disorders including schizophrenia. It is administered in hospital, usually in rooms designated an ECT suite or sometimes (for example if a patient has significant other health problems) in an operating theatre. An ECT suite should have separate rooms for waiting, treatment, and recovery (Royal College of Psychiatrists, 2022).

Qualified staff carry out the procedure involving applying electrodes to the patient's head either temple to temple (bilaterally) or front to back involving one cerebral hemisphere (unilaterally). Staff administer a muscle relaxant and general anaesthetic then induce a voltage causing a direct current to pass through the patient's brain typically for about three to six seconds. Patients usually have several treatments perhaps twice or three times a week for several weeks.

The action of ECT

Bolwig (2011) discusses theories of the action of ECT. A neuroendocrine–diencephalic theory proposes that ECT restores neuroendocrine dysfunction associated with melancholic depression. A combined anatomical–ictal theory (ictal refers to a seizure) argues that seizure activity in the limbic system induces neurotrophic effects crucial for the therapeutic efficacy of ECT. A guidance document by the UK National Institute for Health and Care Excellence (NICE) states of ECT that 'The most prevalent hypothesis is that it causes an alteration in the post-synaptic response to central nervous system neurotransmitters' (NICE, 2003, 2009, 2014, section 3.2) (www.nice.org.uk/guidance/ta59).

A 2012 study indicated that ECT has 'lasting effects' on functional brain architecture. ECT was associated with a decrease in functional connectivity which was accompanied by a 'significant improvement' in depressive symptoms (Perrin et al., 2012).

Conditions treated with ECT

A NICE document (NICE, 2003, 2009, 2014) recommends the use of ECT, 'only to achieve rapid and short-term improvement of severe symptoms.' There should previously have been an 'adequate trial' of other treatments, and they should have been shown to be ineffective, and/or the condition should be considered 'potentially life-threatening, in individuals with catatonia, or a prolonged or severe manic episode' (Ibid., section 1.1). Current evidence does not allow recommending, 'the general use of ECT in the management of schizophrenia.' In the United Kingdom, in current clinical practice, ECT is a treatment choice for people with, 'depressive illness, catatonia and mania.' Also, it is 'occasionally used to treat schizophrenia' (Ibid., section 2.10).

The Mayo Clinic (2018) notes the use of ECT with severe depression especially when accompanied by psychosis, a desire to commit suicide or refusal to eat; treatment resistant depression; severe mania; catatonia; and 'agitation and aggression in people with dementia' (Ibid.).

Contemporary positive findings for the efficacy of ECT

In contrast to findings from some earlier studies for ECT (discussed later) is a more recent controlled study involving treatment resistant schizophrenia. Chanpattana and colleagues (1999) compared the efficacy of continuation treatment with flupentixol alone, continuation ECT alone, and combined continuation of both. Patients with treatment resistant schizophrenia responded to acute combination treatment with ECT and antipsychotics. This was more effective in preventing relapse than ECT or antipsychotics alone.

Petrides and Braga (2009, pp. 297–298) cite open studies and chart reviews of more than 850 patients. These indicate that combination ECT and antipsychotics is more effective than antipsychotics or ECT alone, especially for patients who failed previous treatments with antipsychotics. They include studies by Suzuki and colleagues (2006) and Ucok and Cakr (2006).

More broadly, the Royal College of Psychiatry (2022) reported that 'in 2018–2019, 68% of people who had been treated with ECT were "much improved" or "very much improved" at the end of treatment (1,361 courses out of a total of 2,004). Some of these people were reported as showing no change in their condition and for a very few (1%) it was reported that their condition worsened.

Criticisms of the efficacy of ECT

Negative and emotive colouring of the earliest work on ECT

Petrides and Braga (2009) describe the first use of electricity to cause convulsions. They explain that, in Rome, Ugo Cerletti and Lucio Bini (Cerletti's assistant) performed experiments using electricity. They carried out 'a series of studies in animals.' In 1938, they used the technique on humans for the first time, their first patient being, diagnosed with schizophrenia. He was showing 'agitation, disorganised speech replete with neologisms, and delusional ideas.' The patient 'recovered completely after 11 treatments' (Ibid., p. 290). In brief, initial studies involved animals, the first patient was diagnosed with schizophrenia, and the treatment was successful.

Now consider a dissenting view of the same events. We are told that Ugo Cerletti experimented initially with dogs. He placed the electrodes, 'in the mouth and rectum. Many died.' Where did the notion of placing electrodes on the head occur to Cerletti? It was in 'a slaughterhouse where he saw hogs electrocuted via metallic tongs.' He 'found' his first human patient who was 'a homeless man at a railway station' (Read et al., 2013, p. 90).

It is the same account but coloured and emotive so that it conveys distaste of the use of electricity on people. But why is placing electrodes in the mouth and rectum of dogs and that 'many died' relevant to the effectiveness of ECT with people? Why mention a 'slaughterhouse' and 'hogs' unless to suggest Cerletti devalued human life? When Cerletti 'found' his first patient, was he scouring railway stations for 'homeless' subjects? The message seems to be if this was the foundation of ECT, today's practitioners must devalue human life. No mention is made that the patient recovered. Rhetoric has displaced argument.

Critics citing of earlier negative studies of ECT efficacy – not recognising its limitations

Read et al. (2013, p. 292) cite comparisons with real and fake ECT in several studies. Taylor and Fleminger (1980) found equal improvement in the two groups but noted that real ECT reduced general pathology more than fake. In the Leicester ECT trial (Brandon et al., 1985) both groups improved on all four measures used. The real ECT group did better on two of the four scales but after six weeks had fallen behind with the fake group performing better on all four measures. Abraham and Kulhara (1987) found that after eight weeks the real and fake ECT groups were similar and that any advantage was lost over time. An Indian study (Sarita and Janakiramaiah, 1998) found no differences in symptom reduction between an ECT and fake ECT group even in the short term.

Early research showed no superiority for ECT compared with anti-psychotics. Carried out in the 1980s, 1960s, and 1950s, such studies preceded the later evolution of diagnostic criteria (*DSMIII*) and research methodology. Researchers have argued that the conclusions must be 'viewed with caution.' Such studies 'suffered from significant methodological flaws.' They had samples of 30 or less so may have lacked the power to detect differences. Most used few ECT sessions because of the ethics of giving patients prolonged use of sham ECT. Problems arise where patients took part at various stages of their illness, and where the studies included those with schizophreniform disorder and patients free of medication. This was because many were particularly responsive to medication which could artificially inflate the response rate in both groups (Petrides and Braga, 2009, pp. 291–292).

Potentially misleading citation of research

Given that the interpretation of early studies on ECT require caution, researchers should make it clear when old studies are cited. Recall that the *Hamilton Depression Rating Scale (HAM-D)* (Hamilton, 1960) is a 17-item instrument completed by a clinician. It measures frequency and intensity of depressive symptoms in individuals with major depressive disorder.

Referring to *HAM-D*, Davies (2014) considers, 'recent reviews of ECT research.' He says that research assessing improvement rates of fake compared with real ECT after six months showed a two-point difference in the Hamilton Scale favouring fake treatment. This suggests that, 'if ECT has any positive effects at all these are largely placebo effects' (Davies, 2014, pp. 211–212, citing Bracken et al., 2012).

On the face of it, the passage by Davies (2014) appears to cite research carried out around the time of the publication of his book. He refers to 'recent reviews'; then describes a piece of research into real versus fake ECT, citing as his source, Bracken et al., 2012. In fact, the source is a broad article critical of some approaches in psychiatry that mentions the research in question, the Northwick Park electroconvulsive therapy trial, carried out in 1980 (Johnstone et al., 1980). Davies citing Bracken et al. as his source rather than the 1980 study directly could misleadingly give the impression that the evidence is recent.

Risk and ECT

Memory impairment

Broadly, people endorsing the use of ECT in certain circumstances, and those flatly opposing it, tend to recognise that it can cause memory impairment, although they may differ in details and interpretation.

Guidance from the National Institute for Clinical Excellence summarises the current situation. It says that ECT may cause short- or long-term memory impairment for past and current events. However, as such cognitive impairment is evident with many mental disorders, it may, 'sometimes be difficult to differentiate the effects of ECT from those associated with the condition itself' (NICE, 2003, 2009, 2014, section 3.5).

Concerning the duration of the effects of ECT on cognitive function, random controlled trials have provided 'limited evidence' suggesting that effects on cognitive function may not persist beyond six months. However, 'this has been inadequately researched' (NICE, 2003, 2009, 2014, section 4.1.6).

Turning to the perceptions of some people receiving ECT, the NICE guidance notes that clear evidence exists of cognitive impairment immediately after and following ECT. This 'may cause considerable distress to those affected' (NICE, 2003, 2009, 2014, section 4.1.6). People differ in the extent of memory loss and their perception of it. Importantly, some individuals find it 'extremely damaging and for them this negates any benefit from ECT' (NICE, 2003, 2009, 2014, section 3.5).

The way that electrodes are placed can reduce the risk of cognitive impairment but at the same time tends to reduce treatment efficacy. Less cognitive impairment occurs in individuals who have electrodes applied unilaterally, and still less if they are placed in the non-dominant hemisphere. Any memory impairment appears to vary between individuals and to be linked to the 'dosage' of ECT. However, 'the relationship with the seizure threshold has not been adequately defined' (NICE, 2003, 2009, 2014, section 4.1.6).

ECT-related deaths: critics use of older research

Read et al. (2013, pp. 97–99) select various studies. These indicate 'significantly higher ECT-related death rates' than official statements given by organisations such as the American Psychiatric Association (Ibid., table 8.1, p. 98). The research mentioned includes a 1980 Scotland study with a death rate of 1/92 and a 2004 USA study showing a death rate of 1/1140. It is concluded that many of the findings depended on those who gave the ECT reporting the deaths (Ibid.).

A supposedly 'more objective measure' was 'accidentally provided' by a study of patients' attitudes by Freeman and Kendall (1980). They proposed to interview 183 people a year after they has received ECT. They found however that 12 had died including four who have committed suicide. Read et al. (2013) note that, 'Counting only the two deaths occurring during ECT, the death rate was one per 91.5' (Ibid., p. 99). How does this supposedly more objective measure compare with other judgements of the evidence?

An example is a document from NICE (2003, 2009, 2014) *Guidance on the use of electroconvulsive therapy: Technology appraisal guidance TA 59*. First published in 2003, the report was updated in 2009 and added to a 'static list review' in 2014. This means that the evidence on which the report is based is revisited when new information appears which might lead to the document being amended and updated. In this sense, the report is current (as at 2022). The guidance states that 'There was no evidence to suggest that the mortality associated with ECT is greater than that associated with minor procedures involving general anaesthetics ...' (Ibid., section 4.1.8).

ECT and 'brain damage': critics use of selected research findings and emotive language

Critics tend to have different interpretations of research than orthodox commentators, and they may use emotive language that adds nothing to evidence or argument.

Read et al. (2013) state that in the 1940s and 1950s post-mortem examinations 'consistently provided evidence of brain damage, including necrosis' (Ibid., p. 96). Carney et al. (2003) found ECT to be an effective short-term treatment for depression. Yet the research is cited as showing that CT scans, 'confirmed frontal lobe atrophy following ECT'

(Read et al., 2013, p. 96). Also, the authors refer to an MRI study which, after controlling for level of depression, found that the number of ECTs 'correlated with reduced grey matter density' (citing Shah et al., 2002). Functional brain impairment has also been documented, as when 'marked deactivation' was noted in several regions of the cortex (citing Schmidt et al., 2008).

But historically, it is suggested, psychiatrists seemingly consider damaging the brain to be beneficial. Freeman (1941, p. 83) in a paper, 'Brain Damaging Therapeutics' is quoted as saying, 'The greater the damage, the more likely the remission of psychotic symptoms,' and perhaps, 'a mentally ill patient can think more clearly and more constructively with less brain in actual operation.' Myerson (1942) is quoted as saying that some of the best cures are 'in those individuals whom one reduces almost to amentia.' Supposedly continuing the same theme Perrin et al. (2012) found the ECT reduces the brain's 'functional connectivity' correcting a supposed 'hyperconnectivity' in depressed people (see Read et al., 2013, pp. 96–97).

An example of the exaggerated and emotive language sometimes used in discussions is that of Davies (2014). He observes that many psychiatrists 'still swear' by the effects of ECT. Also, the claims of success are 'more than offset by the reams of research illustrating ECT's ... responsibility for widespread neurological damage' (Ibid.).

Note that psychiatrists 'swear' by the healing effects of ECT as if they are unflinchingly committed and bound by their views. Reference is made to 'reams' of research as if quantity were decisive. But as we have seen, it is important to take account of the quality of the research as well. Also, ECT is said to be responsible for 'widespread neurological damage.'

However, NICE (2003, 2009, 2014) guidance on ECT states that the deaths associated with the treatment are reported 'not to be in excess of that associated with the administration of a general anaesthetic for minor surgery' (Ibid., section 3.4). Also, NICE looked at six studies that used brain-scanning procedures and found that they did not show evidence 'that ECT causes brain damage' (NICE, 2003, 2009, 2014, section 4.1.8).

Torrey (2019) is blunter in his assessment, seeing ECT as a 'favourite whipping boy for Scientologists and anti-psychiatry advocates' and stating, 'there is no evidence that ECT causes damage to the brain' (Ibid., p. 197).

Conclusion

Decades old personal accounts of positive and negative personal experiences of ECT tend to be polarised, and similar extremes of experience are found on the internet today. A broader current picture of patient perspectives is found in surveys and elsewhere.

ECT involves electrically inducing a generalised seizure without muscular convulsions. Electrodes are applied to the patient's head either bilaterally or unilaterally. Staff give a muscle relaxant and general anaesthetic, then induce a voltage causing a direct current to pass through the patient's brain for about three to six seconds. Treatments may be given perhaps twice or three times a week for several weeks.

Among theories of the action of ECT is that generalised seizures are essential for its therapeutic efficacy. A neuroendocrine–diencephalic explanation proposes that ECT restores neuroendocrine dysfunction associated with melancholic depression. A combined anatomical–ictal theory proposes that seizure activity in the limbic system induces neurotrophic effects essential to ECT's therapeutic efficacy.

ECT is sometimes used to treat schizophrenia, for example for catatonia when other treatments have proved ineffective, and the condition is life threatening. Recent studies showing positive effects of ECT include open studies and chart reviews of more than 850 patients. They indicate that ECT and antipsychotics together are more effective than antipsychotics alone or ECT alone. This is particularly the case for patients failing previous treatments with antipsychotics.

Critics of the efficacy of ECT may present a negative and emotive colouring of descriptions of pioneering work. They may not recognise limitations of some earlier studies showing negative findings of ECT efficacy. This is particularly important where these studies preceded improvements in procedures and monitoring of ECT reflected in modern guidance. Critics may cite potentially misleading reference to dates of research, masking reference to old studies.

Current UK guidance recognises that ECT may cause short- or long-term memory impairment for past and current events. Memory impairment being a feature of many mental health problems it may sometimes be difficult to attribute. Cognitive impairment may occur both immediately after administration of ECT and following a course of therapy, which may distress those affected. For individuals perceiving their memory loss as extremely damaging, any benefit from ECT is negated.

Despite critics' reference to older research, current evaluations conclude that there is no evidence suggesting that the mortality associated with ECT is greater than that of minor procedures using general anaesthetics. In discussing ECT and brain damage, critics tend to have different interpretations of research than more orthodox commentators and may also redundantly use emotive language. Current UK guidance notes that six reviewed studies using brain-scanning techniques provided no evidence that ECT causes brain damage.

Suggested further reading

Griffiths, C. and O'Niell-Kerr (2019) 'Patients', carers', and the public's perspectives on electroconvulsive therapy' *Frontiers of Psychiatry* 10, 304. www.ncbi.nlm.nih.gov/pmc/articles/PMC6514218/

Read, J., Bentall, R., Johnstone, L., Foose, R. and Bracken, P. (2013) 'Electroconvulsive therapy' in Read, J. and Dillon, J. (Eds.) (2nd Edition) *Models of Madness: Psychological, Social and Biological Approaches to Psychosis*. London and New York, Routledge (pp. 90–104).

References

Abraham, K. and Kulhara, P. (1987) 'The efficacy of ECT in the treatment of schizophrenia' *British Journal of Psychiatry* 151, 152–155. https://pubmed.ncbi.nlm.nih.gov/3318990/

Benbow, S. M. and Crentsil, J. (2004) 'Subjective experience of electroconvulsive therapy' *Psychiatric Bulletin* 28, 8, 289–291. https://www.cambridge.org/core/journals/psychiatric-bulletin/article/subjective-experience-of-electroconvulsive-therapy/7F9E09DA2D3BBD35AEDD2F528B46414C

Bolwig, T. G. (2011) 'How does electroconvulsive therapy work? Theories on its mechanism' *Canadian Journal of Psychiatry* 56, 1, 13–18. https://pubmed.ncbi.nlm.nih.gov/21324238/

Bracken, P., Thomas, P., Timimi, S., Asen, E., Behr, G., Beuster, C., Bhunnoo, S. and colleagues (2012) 'Psychiatry beyond the current paradigm' *British Journal of Psychiatry* 201, 430–434. https://pubmed.ncbi.nlm.nih.gov/23209088/

Brandon, S., Cowley, P., McDonald, C., Neville, P., Palmer, R. and Wellstood-Eason, S. (1985) 'Leicester ECT trial' *British Journal of Psychiatry* 146, 177–183. https://www.cambridge.org/core/journals/the-british-journal-of-psychiatry/article/abs/leicester-ect-trial-results-in-schizophrenia/62AF7DDBCE875EF9C51E25159DA5D4E9

Carney, S., Cowen, P., Geddes, J. R. and Goodwin, G. (2003) 'Efficacy and safety of ECT in depressive disorders' *Lancet* 361, 799–808. www.thelancet.com/journals/lancet/article/PIIS0140-6736(03)12705-5/fulltext

Chanpattana, W., Chakrabhand, M. L., Sackheim, H. A., Kitaroonchai, W., Kongsakon, R., Techakasem, P., Buppanharun, W., Tuntirungsee, Y. and Kirdcharoen, N. (1999) 'Continuation ECT in treatment resistant schizophrenia: A controlled study' *J ECT* 15, 3, 178–192 www.pubmed.ncbi.nlm.nih.gov/10492856/

Davies, J. (2014) *Cracked: Why Psychiatry Is Doing More Harm than Good*. London, Icon Books.

Davis, N. (2017) 'What is ECT and how does it work?' *The Guardian* (6 September 2018). www.theguardian.com/society/2017/apr/17/what-is-ect-and-how-does … .

Freeman, C. and Kendall, R. (1980) 'ECT: patients' experiences and attitudes' *British Journal of Psychiatry* 137, 8–16. https://www.cambridge.org/core/journals/the-british-journal-of-psychiatry/article/abs/ect-i-patients-experiences-and-attitudes/5EA1482773BCD3AE8EC295D6B133B418

Freeman, W. (1941) 'Brain damaging therapeutics' *Diseases of the Nervous System* 2, 83.

Griffiths, C. and O'Niell-Kerr (2019) 'Patients', carers', and the public's perspectives on electroconvulsive therapy' *Frontiers of Psychiatry* 10, 304. www.ncbi.nlm.nih.gov/pmc/articles/PMC6514218/

Hamilton, M. (1960) 'A rating scale for depression' *Journal of Neurology, Neurosurgery and Psychiatry* 23, 1, 56–62. https://pubmed.ncbi.nlm.nih.gov/14399272/

Johnstone, E. C., Deakin, J. F. W., Lawler, P., Frith, C. D., Stevens, M. and McPherson, K. (1980) 'The Northwick Park electroconvulsive therapy trial' *Lancet* 2, 1317–1320. https://pubmed.ncbi.nlm.nih.gov/6109147/

Kaliora, S. C., Zervas, I. M. and Papadimitriou, G. N. (2018) 'Electroconvulsive therapy: 80 years of use in psychiatry' *Psychiatriki* 29, 4, 291–302. www.psychiatriki-journal.gr/documents/psychiatry/29.4-GR-2018-291.pdf

Mayo Clinic (2018) *Electroconvulsive Therapy (ECT)* (October 2018). www.mayoclinic.org/tests-procedures/electroconvulsive-therapy/about/pac-20393894

Myerson, A. (1942) 'Fatalities following ECT' *Transactions of the American Neurological Association* 68, 39.

NICE (2003, 2009, 2014) *Guidance on the use of electroconvulsive therapy: Technology appraisal guidance TA 59* (Published 2003, Updated 2009, Static list review 2014). www.nice.org.uk/guidance/ta59

Perrin, J. S., Merz, S., Bennett, D. M., Currie, J., Steele, D. J., Reid, I. C. and Schwartzbauer, C. (2012) 'Electro convulsive therapy reduces frontal cortical connectivity in severe depressive disorder' *Biological Sciences* 109, 14, 5464–5468 (19 March 2012). 10.1073/pnas.1117206109

Petrides, G. and Braga, R. J. (2009) 'Electroconvulsive therapy in schizophrenia' in Kasper, S. and Papadimitriou, G. N. (Eds.) (2nd Edition) *Schizophrenia: Biopsychosocial Approaches and Current Challenges* (Medical Psychiatry Series). New York and London, Informa Healthcare (pp. 290–298).

Rayner, L., Kershaw, K., Hanna, D. and Chaplin, R. (2009) 'The patient perspective of the consent process and side effects of electroconvulsive therapy' *Journal of Mental Health* 18, 5, 379–388. https://www.semanticscholar.org/paper/The-patient-perspective-of-the-consent-process-and-Rayner-Kershaw/ecbd4f50a04c24c34c53279a9d6505ba583a961d

Read, J., Bentall, R., Johnstone, L., Foose, R. and Bracken, P. (2013) 'Electroconvulsive therapy' in Read, J. and Dillon, J. (Eds.) (2nd Edition) *Models of Madness: Psychological, Social and Biological Approaches to Psychosis*. London and New York, Routledge (pp. 90–104).

Read, J., Mosher, L. and Bentall, R. (2013) 'Schizophrenia is not an illness' in Read, J. and Dillon, J. (Eds.) (2nd Edition) *Models of Madness: Psychological, Social and Biological Approaches to Psychosis*. London and New York, Routledge (pp. 3–8).

Royal College of Psychiatrists (2016) 'ECTAS 6th national report. London: Royal College of Psychiatrists' *Centre for Quality Improvement*. Royal College of Psychiatrists.

Royal College of Psychiatrists (2022) *Electroconvulsive Therapy (ECT)*. Royal College of Psychiatrists (March 2022). www.rcpsych.ac.uk/mental-health/treatments-and-wellbeing/ect

Rush, G., McCarron, S. H. and Lucey, J. V. (2007) 'Patient attitudes to electroconvulsive therapy' *Psychiatric Bulletin* 31, 6, 212–214. https://www.cambridge.org/core/journals/psychiatric-bulletin/article/patient-attitudes-to-electroconvulsive-therapy/537F8B620A7AE150FF0E6EA713A110F4

Sarita, E. and Janakiramaiah, N. (1998) 'Efficacy of combined ECT after two weeks of neuroleptics in schizophrenia' *NIMHANS Journal* (October, 243–251). https://www.epistemonikos.org/ar/documents/4b0b573a3b8666d1b0933c6a544c02e-31615c8b7

Schmidt, E. Z., Reininghaus, B., Enzinger, C., Ebner, C., Hofmann, P. and Kapfhammer, H. P. (2008) 'Changes in brain metabolism after ECT' *Journal of Affective Disorders* 106, 203–208. https://pubmed.ncbi.nlm.nih.gov/17662472/

Shah, P. J., Glabus, M. F., Goodwin, G. M. and Ebmeier, K. P. (2002) 'Chronic treatment-resistant depression and right fronto-spatial atrophy' *British Journal of Psychiatry* 180, 434–440. https://pubmed.ncbi.nlm.nih.gov/11983641/

Small, J. G., Milstein, V., Klapper, M., Kellhams, J. J. and Small, I. F. (1982) 'ECT combined with neuroleptics in the treatment of schizophrenia' *Psychopharmacological Bulletin* 18, 1, 34–35.

Smith, A. (2018) What it's like to take your own mum for electric shock treatment. Metro (6 September 2018). www.metro.co.uk/2018/02/20/this-is-how-it-feels-to-take-your-mother-f …

Smith, M., Vogler, J., Zarrouf, F., Sheaves, C. and Jesse, J.(2009) 'Electroconvulsive therapy: The struggles in the decision-making process and the aftermath of treatment' *Issues in Mental Health Nursing* 30, 9, 554–559. https://pubmed.ncbi.nlm.nih.gov/19657869/

Suzuki, K., Awata, S., Takano, T., Ebina, Y., Takamatsu, K., Kajiwara, T., Ito, K., Shindo, T., Funakoshi, S. and Matsuoka, H. (2006) 'Improvement of psychiatric symptoms after electroconvulsive therapy in young adults with intractable first-episode schizophrenia and schizophreniform disorder' *Tohoko Journal of Experimental Medicine* 210, 3, 213–220. www.pubmed.ncbi.nlm.nih.gov/17077598/

Talon, L. (2012) What is having ECT like? *The Guardian* (13 May 2012). www.theguardian.com/society/2012/may/13/what-is-having-ect-like

Taylor, P. and Fleminger, J. (1980) 'ECT for schizophrenia' *Lancet* 1, 380.

Torrey, E. F. (2019) (7th Edition) *Surviving Schizophrenia: A Family Manual.* New York and London, Harper Perennial.

Tracy, N. (2022a) 'Personal ECT Story: ECT Saved My Life' HealthyPlace (4 January 2022). www.healthyplace.com/depression/personal-ect-story-ect-saved-my-life

Tracy, N. (2022b) 'Electroshock Therapy: Harmed by Electric Shock Treatment' HealthyPlace (4 January 2022). www.healthyplace.com/depression/electroschock-therapy-harmed-by-electric-shock-treatment

Ucok, A. and Cakr, S. (2006) 'Electroconvulsive therapy in first episode schizophrenia' *Journal of ECT* 22, 1, 38–42. https://pubmed.ncbi.nlm.nih.gov/16633205/

10

INVOLUNTARY HOSPITALISATION AND TREATMENT

Introduction

This chapter examines the aims of hospitalisation, such as allowing patients to be observed and assessed in a controlled setting, and providing respite for families. I look at provision that can reduce hospitalisation, like coordinated specialty care (CSC) programmes for people with first episode psychosis, and Assertive Community Treatment (ACT) for people with schizophrenia who risk becoming homeless or repeatedly hospitalised. I mention Forensic Assertive Community Treatment (FACT) teams. The chapter considers rehabilitation approaches like 'clubhouses' as community facilities for people who have experienced mental disorders. Family psychoeducation (FPE) and training in illness management is discussed.

I consider therapeutic community provision for people with schizophrenia, touching on their development from the 1960s and examining the Soteria approach. The Open Dialogue system of mental health care is also discussed.

Using the example of state legal rationale in the United States, the chapter outlines legal underpinnings of involuntary commitment of patients to psychiatric settings. I touch on the legal reasons for involuntary hospitalisation and physical restraint.

I look at the 1987 United Nations *Convention against Torture and Other Cruel, Inhuman or Degrading Treatment or Punishment* especially Article 1 section 1. Also described is the 2012 United Nations *Convention on the Rights of Persons With Disabilities*. Article 12 and Article 15. Connected with these conventions, the chapter considers Méndez' 2013 *Report of the Special Rapporteur on Torture and Other Cruel, Inhuman*

DOI: 10.4324/9781003413554-10

or Degrading Treatment or Punishment. This links aspects of psychiatric provision on the one hand, and treatments and torture, and other cruel, inhuman, or degrading treatment of punishment on the other. Méndez' report was depicted as a call for a ban on forced psychiatric treatment including drugging, ECT, psychosurgery, restraint, and seclusion.

However, soon after Méndez' document appeared, the Center for Human Rights and Humanitarian Law: Anti-Torture Initiative (2014) published their own report bringing together a range of contributions concerning Méndez' report. This included rebuttals to which Méndez responded, substantially qualifying what he had earlier said.

I note that the need for involuntary hospitalisation and treatment is recognised in certain circumstances. At the same time, procedures are being examined to ensure that they are fit for purpose, and clinicians and others are seeking safe ways to further reduce involuntary hospitalisation and treatment.

Orthodox and dissenting positions

An orthodox perspective is that hospitalisation is usually necessary for patients with schizophrenia who have the disorder for the first time. Hospitalisation can sometimes be avoided for people who have already been diagnosed and have had a relapse. In these instances, there are 'several possible alternatives' (Torrey, 2019, p. 167). Where the rate of treatment is low, this can be attributed to legal changes making it harder to arrange involuntary hospitalisation and treatment for people having, 'no awareness of their need for treatment' (Ibid., p. 368). Opponents of 'assisted treatment' claim that its effects are 'devastating' whereas studies have found it in the majority of cases to be, 'remarkably benign' (Ibid., p. 271–272). Similarly, it has been found that, when discharged from hospital, most patients said that their admission was 'justified' even though they were hospitalised involuntarily (Gowda et al., 2016, conclusions).

Turning to a dissenting position, it has been said that a simplistic view may be held that, because the person has no insight into their illness, 'they need to be detained and administered medication, by force if necessary' (Cooke, 2017, section 13.1). Reference may be made to a United Nations Special Rapporteur who called for 'a ban on forced psychiatric treatment' which included drugs, ECT, psychosurgery, restraint and seclusion (Cooke, 2017, section 13.5.3). Dissenters may claim that there exists a 'misguided but powerful minority' who proclaim that schizophrenia is an illness requiring drugs, given by force if necessary (Read, Mosher and Bentall, 2013, pp. 4–5). A little used approach known as Soteria is sometimes cited. It rejects a 'disease model' of schizophrenia, 'professionally acquired' views and practices, and antipsychotic medication (Mosher and Boler, 2013, p. 364).

Reasons for hospitalisation

Several reasons for hospitalisation have been identified. It allows mental health professionals to observe patients in a 'controlled setting' (Torrey, 2019, p. 158). Laboratory tests can be carried out to exclude other medical illnesses that might be causing the observed symptoms. Psychological testing can be done. Medication may be started in a setting where trained staff can watch for any side effects. At the same time the patient's family, if they had a difficult time with the patient in the days before admission, get some respite (Ibid.).

Also, hospitalisation may protect the patient from harming themselves or others, for example because of hallucinations ordering them to do so. Hospital facilities for group meetings, occupational therapy, and recreational activities can allow the patient to meet others with similar problems and perhaps recognise that they are not alone (Ibid.).

Provision which may reduce hospitalisation

Coordinated Specialty Care (CSC) refers to programmes for people with first episode psychosis. They involve a team of health professionals and specialists delivering a comprehensive package of provision such as psychotherapy, medication management, case management, support for employment and education, and family education and help. Working together, the patient and the team, make treatment decisions, as far as possible involving family members (National Institute of Mental Health, accessed 2021). CSC can reduce the chance of relapse that can lead to rehospitalisation.

In the United States, Assertive Community Treatment (ACT) is designed for people with schizophrenia who risk becoming homeless or repeatedly hospitalised. A multidisciplinary team offer direct service provision, frequent patient contact, low patient to staff ratios, and community outreach (National Institute of Mental Health, May 2020 revision, paraphrased). ACT involves teams of around 10 mental health professionals and paraprofessionals responsible for 100–150 people with severe mental disorders including schizophrenia. A team member attending to clinical, housing and rehabilitation needs offers 24/7 on call coverage.

ACT treatment team members meet patients, often elsewhere than the professional's offices. Medication is delivered directly to patients. Team members who may see the same patients over many years, proactively seek them out for their follow-up care (Torrey, 2019, p. 229). If the individual is hospitalised or jailed, the ACT member visits them, liaising with whoever oversees their treatment (Ibid.). Randomised trials indicate that ACT patients have lower rates of hospitalisation, and that patients and their families highly value the provision. Forensic Assertive Community Treatment (FACT) teams have been developed for individuals with serious mental disorders who have been charged with criminal offences.

Rehabilitation can reduce rehospitalisation. In the United States, 'clubhouses' are community facilities for people who have had mental disorders. Open seven days a week, the clubhouse enables members to meet for social and educational activities. Most link with housing programmes through which members share apartments or houses. Participants are strongly encouraged to take any prescribed medication. Regarding vocational rehabilitation, members are expected to join work teams that maintain the clubhouse – cleaning, preparing lunch, and answering the telephone. Formal vocational training is offered, helping members to find work.

Family psychoeducation (FPE) and training in illness management recognises the importance of family involvement in treating and caring for people with schizophrenia. FPE offers 'structured psychotherapeutic interventions' involving the person with schizophrenia and their family as 'partners in care.' Trained practitioners collaboratively share information and provide training in 'coping, communication, and problem-solving skills.' Evidence points to reduced relapse rates for schizophrenia. Despite practice guideline recommendations, FPE is not widely available worldwide. This might be improved by 'systematic approaches to practice change and tiered approaches to family service delivery' (Harvey, 2018, abstract).

Alternative provision

In the 1960s and 1970s, a residential schizophrenia treatment centre associated with psychiatrist R D. Laing opened in London (Chapman, 2021). Workers tried to understand schizophrenia non-medically, to avoid antipsychotic medication as the first resort, and provide high levels of support (Calton et al., 2008).

An approach termed 'Soteria' offers small community-based therapeutic settings of mainly lay front-line staff with professionals available. Antipsychotic medication is avoided or limited and taken voluntarily. Staff try to understand a person's experiences of psychosis (Calton et al., 2008). Two Soteria projects in the United States and one in Switzerland were evaluated (Calton et al., 2008). While Soteria seemed as effective as orthodox hospital-based treatment, it remained, 'an intriguing, but in many ways still experimental approach' (Ibid.). Such therapeutic communities represent not just alternatives to hospitalisation, but an alternative approach to overall treatment.

Developed in Finland in the 1980s, Open Dialogue is a system of mental health care. It proposes a therapeutic and philosophical approach to being 'with people' in crisis. It seeks to organise health services to increase the chances of them responding accordingly, and in a timely way. This often involves a network meeting in the community in which the person of concern and significant others participate (Putman and Martindale, 2022).

Having discussed provision that can reduce hospitalisation and re-hospitalisation, or that offers alternatives, we now turn to situations where involuntary hospitalisation and treatment are considered necessary.

Involuntary hospitalisation and treatment

Where people with schizophrenia lack insight into their condition and do not accept that they may hurt themselves or others, it may be necessary to commit them, 'to psychiatric treatment settings against their will' (Torrey, 2019, pp. 160–161).

In the United States, laws for committing psychiatric patients are state laws not federal ones. Legal rationale is twofold. Firstly, 'parens patriae' is the right of the state to act like a parent to protect disabled people. The second legal justification is the right of the state to protect people from someone who is dangerous.

Commitment may be 'emergency' or 'long-term.' Emergency commitments tend to be about 72 hours. Hospitalisation may be necessary to protect a patient who may try to injure themselves or others owing to their illness. A hospital may use a locked ward for 'acutely agitated patients.' Additional equipment may be required like ankle restraints or a special jacket keeping the arms next to the body. None of these steps should be necessary for more than a few hours, 'if the person is being properly medicated' (Torrey, 2019, p. 158).

We now turn to examining two United Nation conventions, and a report which referred extensively to them. The report drew links between certain involuntary psychiatric provision and torture and other cruel, inhuman, or degrading treatment. In the summaries below, some paraphrasing has been used to try to give the sense of the documents. As with legal and similar documents, the original text should be consulted for the precise wording.

United Nations *Convention against Torture and Other Cruel, Inhuman or Degrading Treatment or Punishment* (adopted 1987)

In the United Nations *Convention against Torture and Other Cruel, Inhuman or Degrading Treatment or Punishment*, adopted in 1987, Article 1 section 1 defines torture as, 'any act by which severe pain or suffering, whether physical or mental, is intentionally inflicted on a person' for certain purposes.

These purposes (regarding the person being tortured or a third person) involve obtaining information or a confession, punishment for an act committed or suspected of having been committed, intimidation or coercion, or for 'any reason based on discrimination of any kind.' It is specified that the pain or suffering is inflicted by or instigated with the consent or acquiescence of a person acting in an official capacity. It excludes that 'arising only from, inherent in, or incidental to lawful sanctions.'

UN *Convention on the Rights of Persons with Disabilities* 2012

Article 12

The United Nations (2012) *Convention on the Rights of Persons with Disabilities* Article 12 has five sections concerning what states ('states parties') should do and not do. They should reaffirm the rights of people with disabilities to be recognised in all places as, 'persons before the law' (section 1). States parties recognise that disabled people have legal capacity equally with others in 'all aspects of life' (section 2). They should take suitable steps to give access by people having disabilities to support that they may need in 'exercising their legal capacity' (section 3).

Section 4 provides that States Parties ensure that measures concerning the exercise of legal capacity provide safeguards to stop abuse in line with international human rights law. These safeguards must make sure that measures to do with exercising legal capacity, respect the 'rights, will and preferences' of the person. They should involve no conflict of interest or undue influence and should be proportional and fitted to the circumstances of the disabled person. They should, apply for the briefest time possible and be subject to regular review by an appropriate authority or judicial body. In section 5, the convention specifies that States Parties shall take suitable measures to ensure the equal right of disabled people in relation to property, the control their own finances, and related matters.

Article 15

Article 15 of the Convention (United Nations, 2012) concerning torture or cruel, inhuman, or degrading treatment or punishment states that no one shall be subjected to such treatment or punishment. Without free consent, no one should be subjected to, 'medical or scientific experimentation' (section 1). States parties must take all effective measures to make sure that disabled people, like others, are not subjected to the specified treatment or punishment (section 2).

Criticism that coercive treatment may constitute torture – a slippery redefinition of 'torture'

In 2013, a report was published linking the two UN conventions just outlined. This *Special Rapporteur on Torture and Other Cruel, Inhuman or Degrading Treatment or Punishment* (Méndez, 2013) highlights aspects of Article 12 of the *UN Convention on the Rights of Persons with Disabilities*. This recognises that all persons should enjoy 'legal capacity' in all aspects of life on an 'equal basis with others' (see also Freeman, Kolappa, and de Almeida, 2015). Méndez (2013) argues that contrary to 'medical necessity' and 'best interest' doctrines, this implies that coercive treatment relates to torture, and demands that coercive measures be abolished. He recommends that national policies should ban coercive treatment and that laws or policies related to 'substituted decision making' be replaced with 'supported decision making.' This challenges the conception that impaired capacity is central to decisions made against a patient's will.

Forensic psychiatrist Paul Appelbaum, a drafter of the American Psychiatric Association's response to Méndez' report, rejected the redefinition of torture. Appelbaum stated that the report contained much, 'slippery language.' He argued that all the recommendations in the Méndez report followed from the initial position to redefine torture to include 'involuntary hospitalization or treatment when people have been found incompetent to make decisions or are dangerous to self or others' (Levin, 2014).

The Center for Human Rights and Humanitarian Law: Anti-Torture Initiative (2013) published their response to Méndez' document. Included was a joint statement by Lieberman, Levin, and Ruiz (respectively the President, American Psychiatric Association, CEO and Medical Director American Psychiatric Association, and President World Psychiatric Association). There were extensive rebuttals of much of Méndez' earlier 2013 report.

Key paragraphs of the Méndez' Report 2013 and rebuttals

Méndez' (2013) report raised key issues to which the joint statement provided by Lieberman, Levin and Ruiz (2013) responded paragraph by paragraph. I provide a selection below. To avoid constant repetition of reference to these three authors, I sometimes refer to their responses as being from 'psychiatric bodies.'

Criticism that medically indicated involuntary treatment may constitute torture – overlooks protective aspects

Méndez (2013, paragraph 32) states that any treatment without a therapeutic purpose constitutes, at least, 'ill-treatment.' The discriminatory character of forced psychiatric interventions involving people with psychosocial disabilities, satisfies intent and purpose required under Article 1 of the Convention against Torture. This is despite claims of good intentions by medical professionals.

Lieberman, Levin and Ruiz (2013) maintain that medically indicated involuntary treatment used in appropriate circumstances can restore the 'functional and decisional capacity' of people experiencing severe mental disorders. In doing this, such treatment can protect the affected person and others from 'the behavioural consequences of their conditions.'

Criticism that the doctrine of medical necessity hinders protection – overlooks that it helps ensure appropriate use of involuntary treatment

Méndez (2013, paragraph 35) maintains, the doctrine of medical necessity gets in the way of protection from 'arbitrary abuses in health-care settings.' Consequently, treatment that violates the terms of the Convention on the Rights of Persons with Disabilities, through coercion or discrimination, cannot be legitimated or justified as medical necessity.

Psychiatric bodies accepted that medical necessity is insufficient alone 'to justify involuntary treatment of capable persons.' However, the doctrine of medical necessity is essential to ensuring that involuntary treatment is used only when it is appropriate and when other interventions are unlikely to succeed.

Criticism that solitary confinement and restraint may constitute torture – justified if it is the only way to prevent harm

Méndez (2013, paragraph 63) rejects therapeutic justification in psychiatric institutions for solitary confinement and 'prolonged restraint' of disabled persons. Both these measures may 'constitute torture and ill-treatment' (A/63/175, paragraphs 55–56). Méndez states that in psychiatric and social care institutions, there should be an 'absolute ban' on all measures that are coercive and not consented to. These measures include 'restraint and solitary confinement' of people with psychological or intellectual disabilities. Using restraint and seclusion can lead to further non-consensual treatment like, 'forced medication and electroshock procedures' (Méndez, 2013, paragraph 63).

Lieberman, Levin and Ruiz (2013) state that for psychotic patients trying to severely injure themselves or others, restraint may be 'the only way to prevent severe injury' to the patient and protect other people. They note that restrained patients must be monitored carefully, and that restraints should be in place for the shortest time possible.

The view that institutionalising legislation should be abolished – it can be life saving

Méndez (2013, paragraph 68) calls for abolishing laws that authorise the 'institutionalisation' of disabled people because of their disability without their giving 'free and informed consent.' This includes institutionalisation as the provision of treatment and care, and where it is based on the chances of the person being a danger to themselves or others. It applies to cases where legislation links the grounds of care, treatment, and public security to 'mental illness' (A/HRC/10/48, paragraphs 48, 49).

Lieberman, Levin and Ruiz (2013) oppose abolishment of institutionalisation legislation, saying that hospitalising people with psychiatric disorders, 'can be lifesaving, and result in restoring a person with the ability to direct his or her own life.'

Criticism that severity of mental illness should not justify deprivation of liberty – it can be appropriate to avoid suffering

For Méndez (2013, paragraph 69), depriving liberty owing to mental illness is unjustified if it is based on discrimination or prejudice against people with disabilities. The severity of the mental disorder of itself is not sufficient to justify detention. The state must also demonstrate that detention is needed to 'protect the safety of the person or of others.' Except in an emergency, the individual should not be deprived of liberty unless 'of unsound mind.' Because detention in a psychiatric context may lead to non-consensual psychiatric treatment, the mandate states that deprivation of liberty might fall under the scope of the *Convention against Torture* (A/63/175, paragraph 65). This could arise when the grounds for depriving liberty are those of disability, and when it 'inflicts severe pain or suffering.'

Lieberman, Levin and Ruiz (2013) argue that the severe impairment and suffering because of mental illness can be an 'appropriate basis' for using involuntary hospitalisation.

Méndez' response to Lieberman, Levin, and Ruiz

Méndez responded to points raised by Lieberman, Levin, and Ruiz (2013, pp. 151–153). His responses effectively reduced the perceived influence of his report and any notion that its contents represented international views or consensus.

In the report, Méndez acknowledges that his wording' had led to misunderstandings. Indeed, the document did not intend to propose an absolute ban on non-consensual interventions under any and all circumstances. Méndez accepted that his proposal largely coincides with the highest professional standards of the psychiatric profession as reflected in the policy statements provided to him by the psychiatric bodies.

Specifically, Méndez stated that there were no plans to continue the discussion or to adopt the report. Reports from mandate-holders like Méndez are 'not submitted for adoption by the Council.' They are only intended for discussion.

Méndez regretted that some 'inartful wording' led to some of his statements being misunderstood. Also, some passages could be 'legitimately read' as contradicting other sections. He did not intend to call for an 'absolute ban on non-consensual interventions ... under any and all circumstances.' Méndez points out that he mentions that involuntary detention and treatment *is* legitimate in certain circumstances. These are if it intends to stop patient harming themselves or others, and as long as it is for the 'limited time and scope necessary to prevent such harm.'

Misunderstanding of Méndez report

What seemed to link the treatment of psychiatric patients (viewed through the lens of the rights of disabled people) with torture and other cruel, inhuman, or degrading treatment or punishment turned out not to do so. Unsurprisingly, given Méndez original report and the subsequent major qualifying of his position, this was not always understood.

A report published by the British Psychological Society stated, 'The United Nations Special Rapporteur on Torture and Other Cruel, Inhuman or Degrading Treatment has called for a ban on forced psychiatric treatment including drugging, ECT (electro-convulsive therapy), psychosurgery, restraint and seclusion' (Cooke, 2017, section 13.5.3).

Yet as Méndez (2013) had stated, he did not intend to propose such an 'absolute ban' in, 'any and all circumstances.' Also, he mentioned that such involuntary detention and treatment is 'legitimate' when intended to stop a patient seriously harming themselves or others and is for a justified limited time (Ibid.).

However, while seeming calls for banning involuntary hospitalisation and treatment were being clarified so that they did not call for any such ban, more sober approaches were being considered. These were intended to further reduce the use of involuntary hospitalisation and treatment conversant with patient and public safety.

Further reducing involuntary hospitalisation and treatment

While the need for involuntary hospitalisation and treatment is recognised in certain circumstances, researchers and clinicians are examining procedures to ensure that these interventions are fit for purpose. They are seeking ways to reduce involuntary steps where these do not compromise safety. One reason for reviewing numbers and analysing them is to ensure that psychiatrists and others do not have an unrecognised bias relating to class, gender, or race for example that could distort referrals.

Chieze et al. (2021) note that coercion is frequent in psychiatry. It requires legal and ethical justification as it overrides some rights of patients including 'liberty of movement and decision-making.' The authors set out the ethical elements used in the literature to justify or reject coercive measures that limit freedom of movement. These are involuntary hospitalisation, restraint, and seclusion. Clinicians should, the authors conclude, before using such coercive measures, evaluate all the relevant ethical aspects of the situation. They should, seek alternatives that treat the patient's well-being and rights more respectfully. Where coercive measures are decided after a well-considered process of evaluation, they are more likely to be 'adequate, understood, and accepted by patients and care-givers' (Ibid.).

One strategy in seeking to reduce coercion is the use of 'advance statements.' These record information on an individual's treatment refusal, treatment preferences and personal care instructions. Their content includes medical treatment instructions, medical preferences, medication refusals (with reasons), preference/refusal of ECT, and preferred methods of de-escalating crisis (Jankovic, Richards and Priebe, 2010, box 2).

Jankovic, Richards and Priebe (2010) reviewed literature on advance statements and describe their use, advantages, disadvantages, and barriers to their implementation. They note that as well as information on treatment refusals, advance statements give information about other matters. These matters like treatment preferences and personal care instructions are not legally binding, but they should inform decisions made about treatment. Advance statements, the authors suggest, could 'reduce coercion and improve service users' satisfaction with treatment' (Ibid.).

More recently, a review and meta-analysis was carried out on interventions to reduce compulsory psychiatric admissions (De Jong et al., 2016). In adult psychiatric patients, the meta-analysis of randomised clinical trials on advance statements showed a 23% reduction in compulsory admissions. This was both statistically significant and clinically relevant. A similar analysis on community treatment orders, compliance enhancement, and integrated treatment showed no evidence of such a reduction (Ibid.).

Also important are consistency in the use of procedures. In Bangalore, India, researchers carried out a hospital-based observational study of patient experiences of involuntary admission and treatment. It involved

76 people with schizophrenia admitted under the Mental Health Act 1987. Within three days of admission, demographic and clinical assessments and experiences of coercion were completed. Just before discharge, an assessment of 67 patients was made. At discharge, most patients reported that their admissions were justified. The authors stated that the study underlines the need for a standardised rule of conduct based coercive practice in psychiatry' (Gowda et al., 2016).

Conclusion

Hospitalisation allows patients to be observed and assessed in a controlled setting and can provide respite for families. Provision that can reduce hospitalisation includes coordinated specialty care (CSC) programmes for people with first episode psychosis, Assertive Community Treatment (ACT) for people with schizophrenia who risk becoming homeless or repeatedly hospitalised, and Forensic Assertive Community Treatment (FACT) teams for individuals with serious mental disorder charged with criminal offences. Other provision that can reduce hospitalisation are rehabilitation for example clubhouses which are community facilities for people who have had mental disorders, and family psychoeducation and training in illness management. Therapeutic community alternatives to hospitalisation for people with schizophrenia include the Soteria approach. The Open Dialogue system of mental health care offers community alternatives.

In the United States, legal underpinnings for involuntary commitment of patients to psychiatric settings includes state legal rationale setting out reasons for hospitalisation and physical restraint.

The United Nations *Convention against Torture and Other Cruel, Inhuman or Degrading Treatment or Punishment* of 1987 Article 1 section 1 defines torture. In the United Nations (2012) *Convention on the Rights of Persons With Disabilities*, Article 12 'Equal recognition before the law' sets how 'States Parties' should act in relation to 'disabled people' while Article 15 concerns, 'Freedom from torture or cruel, inhuman or degrading treatment or punishment.'

The 2013 Special Rapporteur on Torture and Other Cruel, Inhuman or Degrading Treatment or Punishment draws on the United Nations *Convention against Torture and Other Cruel, Inhuman or Degrading Treatment or Punishment* of 1987 and the United Nations 2012 *Convention on the Rights of Persons With Disabilities.*

Méndez' report makes connections between aspects of psychiatric provision and treatments and torture, and other cruel, inhuman or degrading treatment of punishment. Subsequently, the Center for Human Rights and Humanitarian Law: Anti-Torture Initiative (2014) published their own report bringing together a range of contributions concerning Méndez' report including rebuttals. Méndez' clarified and modified much of what he had said and.pointed out that the report was for discussion purposes.

Involuntary hospitalisation and treatment are needed in certain circumstances. Researchers and clinicians are seeking to ensure that procedures are fit for purpose. Safe ways of reducing involuntary hospitalisation and treatment are being developed, for example the use of advance statements.

Suggested further reading

Lieberman, J., Levin, S. and Ruiz, P. (2013) 'Joint Statement from the American Psychiatric Association and the World Psychiatric Association' in Center for Human Rights and Humanitarian Law: Anti-Torture Initiative (2013) *Torture in Healthcare Settings: Reflections on the Special Report on Torture's 2013 Thematic Report* American University Washington College of Law - Center for Human Rights and Humanitarian Law (December 2013) (pp. 141–146).

Méndez, J. E. (2013) *Report of the Special Rapporteur on Torture and Other Cruel, Inhuman or Degrading Treatment or Punishment.* New York, United Nations, Human Rights Council. http://www.hr-dp.org/files/2013/10/28/A. HRC.22.53SpecialRappReport.2013.pdf

References

Calton, T., Ferriter, M., Huband, N. and Spandler, H. (2008) 'A systematic review of the Soteria paradigm for the treatment of people diagnosed with schizophrenia' *Schizophrenia Bulletin* 34, 1, 181–192. https://www.ncbi.nlm.nih.gov/pmc/articles/PMC2632384/

Center for Human Rights and Humanitarian Law: Anti-Torture Initiative (2013) *Torture in Healthcare Settings: Reflections on the Special Report on Torture's 2013 Thematic Report.* American University Washington College of Law - Center for Human Rights and Humanitarian Law (December 2013).

Chapman, A. (2021) 'Dwelling in strangeness: Accounts of the Kingsley Hall Community, London (1965–1970), established by R. D. Laing' *Journal of Medical Humanities* 42, 471–494. https://doi.org/10.1007/s10912-020-09656-0

Chieze, M., Clavien, C., Kaiser, S. and Hurst, S., (2021) 'Coercive measures in psychiatry: A review of ethical arguments' *Frontiers of Psychiatry* 12 (December 2021). https://www.frontiersin.org/articles/10.3389/fpsyt.2021.790886/full

Cooke, A. (Ed.) (2017) *Understanding Psychosis and Schizophrenia: Why people sometimes hear voices, believe things that others find strange, or appear out of touch with reality, and what can help.* British Psychological Society Division of Clinical Psychology/Canterbury Christchurch University.

De Jong, M. H., Kamperman, A. M., Oorschot, M., Preibe, S., Bramer, W., van der Sand, R., Van Gool, A. R. and Mulder, C. (2016) 'Interventions to reduce compulsory psychiatric admissions: A systematic review and meta-analysis' *JAMA Psychiatry* 73, 7, 657–664. https://pubmed.ncbi.nlm.nih.gov/27249180/

Freeman, M. C., Kolappa, K., de Almeida, J. M. C., Kleinman, A., Makhashvili, N., Phakathi, S., Saraceno, B. and Thornicroft, G. (2015) 'Reversing hard-won victories in the name of human rights: A critique of the General Comment on Article 12 of the UN Convention on the Rights of Persons with Disabilities' *Lancet Psychiatry* 2, 844–850.

Gowda, G. S., Kondapuram, N., Kumar, C. N. and Badamath, S. (2016) 'Involuntary admission and treatment experiences of persons with schizophrenia: Implications for the Mental Health Care Bill 2016' *Asian Journal of Psychiatry* 29 (3–7 October). https://pubmed.ncbi.nlm.nih.gov/29061422/

Harvey, C. (2018) 'Family psychoeducation for people living with schizophrenia and their families' *British Journal of Psychology Advances* 24, 9–19. https://www.researchgate.net/publication/322345244_Family_psychoeducation_for_people_living_with_schizophrenia_and_their_families

Jankovic, J., Richards, F. and Priebe, S. (2010) 'Advance statements in adult mental health' *Advances in Psychiatric Treatment* 16, 6, 448–455, November (Published online by Cambridge University Press: 2 January 2018). https://www.cambridge.org/core/journals/advances-in-psychiatric-treatment/article/advance-statements-in-adult-mental-health/8B19643F96B6F08D3D1CEAD6438BBD76

Levin, A. (2014) 'UN report says common psychiatric practices amount to 'torture' *Psychiatric News* (American Psychiatric Association 25 April 2014). https://psychnews.psychiatryonline.org/doi/full/10.1176/appi.pn.2014.5a11

Lieberman, J., Levin, S. and Ruiz, P. (2013) 'Joint statement from the American Psychiatric Association and the World Psychiatric Association' in Center for Human Rights and Humanitarian Law: Anti-Torture Initiative (2013) *Torture in Healthcare Settings: Reflections on the Special Report on Torture's 2013 Thematic Report*, American University Washington College of Law - Center for Human Rights and Humanitarian Law (December 2013) (pp. 141–146).

Méndez, J. E. (2013) *Report of the Special Rapporteur on Torture and Other Cruel, Inhuman or Degrading Treatment or Punishment*. New York, United Nations, Human Rights Council. http://www.hr-dp.org/files/2013/10/28/A.HRC.22.53SpecialRappReport.2013.pdf

Mosher, L. and Boler, J. (2013) 'Non-hospital, non-medication interventions in first episode psychosis' in Read, J. and Dillon, J. (Eds.) (2nd Edition) *Models of Madness: Psychological, Social and Biological Approaches to Psychosis*. London and New York, Routledge (pp. 361–377).

National Institute of Mental Health (accessed 2021) *Coordinated specialty care (CSC)*. https://www.nimh.nih.gov/

Putman, N. and Martindale, B. (Eds.) (2022) *Open Dialogue for Psychosis* (The International Society for Psychological and Social Approaches to Psychosis Book Series). London, Routledge.

Read, J., Mosher, L. and Bentall, R. (2013) 'Schizophrenia is not an illness' in Read, J. and Dillon, J. (Eds.) (2nd Edition) *Models of Madness: Psychological,*

Social and Biological Approaches to Psychosis. London and New York, Routledge (pp. 3–8).

Torrey, E. F. (2019) (7th Edition) *Surviving Schizophrenia: A Family Manual.* New York and London, Harper Perennial.

United Nations (2012) *Convention on the Rights of Persons With Disabilities.* United Nations.

11

CHALLENGES AND CRITICISMS

Introduction

In this chapter (and the next) are drawn together points arising in previous ones. Here, I reiterate examples of the challenges relating to schizophrenia. These are schizophrenia's weak validity and reliability along with the permeability of psychosis; and research and claims associated with pharmaceutical companies that suggest caution. That these issues are challenges is largely agreed by orthodox practitioners and dissenters, although the responses to them may differ.

After this, I review types of dissenting criticisms of schizophrenia, pointing out their weaknesses. I first cover overstatement, emotive language, euphemism, and other rhetorical devices.

Examples of overstatement are evident in criticism that schizophrenia is unscientific paralleling astrology, a negative depiction of genetic research, and the presentation of evidence that antipsychotics are implicated in brain anomalies in schizophrenia. Other instances are discussion of the possible role of childhood trauma in schizophrenia, and Faustian allusions to the sedating effects of antipsychotics.

Emotive language is exemplified by the view that schizophrenia was 'invented,' criticisms of a medical view of schizophrenia, scepticism about the efficacy of ECT, and discussion of ECT and brain damage. Instances of euphemism arise also in maintaining that schizophrenia was invented; and proposing continua as an alternative to categorisation. Other rhetoric involves the laudatory presentation of supportive evidence, and critics misrepresenting an orthodox position towards antipsychotics.

DOI: 10.4324/9781003413554-11

Another type of dissenting criticism identified by this chapter concerns conflicting and weak evidence. Examples are weaknesses of using symptoms for identification and assessment instead of categorisation, criticisms that the 'medical model' is pessimistic, and proposing that understanding schizophrenia as an illness is just another theory. Further instances are claims that biogenetic causal beliefs involve negative attitudes while psychosocial beliefs involve positive attitudes, mistrustful presentation of evidence of research involving drug companies, and claims that those with schizophrenia in developing countries do better with less access to antipsychotics.

Challenges facing the orthodox view of schizophrenia

Challenges confront an orthodox perspective of schizophrenia. These are pointed out by dissenters and largely accepted by orthodox practitioners. Generally, orthodoxy considers that the challenges can be met while dissenters believe that the obstacles that arise are insurmountable. A few examples should illustrate.

Challenges: schizophrenia's weak validity and reliability; and the permeability of psychosis

Critics maintain that the category of schizophrenia is not valid enough or sufficiently reliable to ensure secure identification. Schizophrenia defined operationally, is encroached by neighbouring entities. It lacks a single origin. Many possible causal indications exist, for example in brain structure and functioning, but are not always present. Psychotic disorders are defined by their symptoms, which can mislead because different disorders can produce the same symptoms. Also, no single symptom definitively identifies schizophrenia. In practice, indications may be difficult to recognise because schizophrenia is episodic and is latent at the time of assessment. Diagnosis is dependent upon a psychiatrist's partly subjective judgement which is based on observations of the individual.

Issues arise about the extent to which psychosis, included under the construct of schizophrenia, lacks characteristics of a categorical entity. This is reflected by diagnostic problems when assessing cases jointly presenting symptoms of psychosis and mood. It is also evident in the high comorbidity of schizophrenia with other mental disorders, and difficulties in diagnosing sub-threshold psychotic states. Although schizophrenia is seen as categorical, psychotic illness appears more permeating. This suggests avoiding too rigid a separation of mental disorders, and questioning the suitability of a categorical approach for studying psychosis.

Challenges concerning the validity and reliability of schizophrenia and the permeability of psychosis pose a key choice. Clinicians, researchers, and others either abandon the construct of schizophrenia, or develop and refine it based on evidence as it stands currently and as it emerges in the future. Dissenters favour ditching, while orthodox practitioners support refining.

Challenges – research and claims associated with pharmaceutical companies invite caution

Concerns about the use of medication include worries about the involvement of large pharmaceutical companies. This is expressed not only by some critics, but also by a number of orthodox practitioners.

There is a worry that the impartiality of some psychiatrists and groups to evaluate the efficacy of certain drugs may be impaired by too close an association with pharmaceutical companies. High financial benefits to drug companies and aggressive marketing also create unease. Accusations that some pharmaceutical firms distort claims of drug benefits damages their reputation.

Typical of such views are the comments of Davies (2014) who notes that drug firms can be 'notoriously secretive.' He states that in the past, some of these companies have concealed how drugs are developed and put on the market. They have also he affirms, concealed negative trials (Ibid., p. 88). Davies gives an account of the drug company AstraZeneca and their discovery in early 2000 that its latest research into its own drug Seroquel indicated that it was not as effective as a rival drug Haldol (Ibid., p. 148).

In response, the company adopted 'cherry picking' publishing only selected data from clinical trials. The company, Davies maintains, did not admit that, after a year taking Seroquel, patients experienced more relapses and had poorer ratings on different scales assessing symptoms than did patients taking Haldol. Neither was it mentioned that patients gained weight (on average 5 kg) which increased the risk of diabetes. Rather than this, the company focused on, 'one shred of positive data' about Seroquel doing a little better on some measures of cognition (Ibid., pp. 150–151).

Davies (2014) states that this approach eventually backfired. Many people taking Seroquel were experiencing unpleasant adverse effects. Around 17,500 of them were claiming officially that the firm had 'lied about the risks of the drug.' These claims were shown to be valid when in 2010 when AstraZeneca paid £125 million 'to settle a class action out of court for defrauding the public' (Ibid., p. 152).

Goldacre (2012) presents broader criticism expressing concern about the process of getting pharmaceuticals licensed for clinical purposes, then maximising their use by physicians and patients. This has compromised study design and the open sharing of data about study results. National drug regulatory organisations have not always ensured that studies have focused on the right groups of patients, that cost, and effectiveness are fully considered, and that value is added to existing treatments.

I suggested earlier that criticism of some pharmaceutical companies is shared by those holding orthodox and dissenting positions. However, dissenters tend to be more sceptical about proposals to put matters right. Among efforts to improve the situation is the development of new codes of industry practice, ensuring open-access disclosure by prescribers and clinical trialists who get industry funding, and a requirement of open access to full clinical trial data.

Criticisms of orthodox positions on schizophrenia

Among dissenting criticisms of orthodox views on schizophrenia are those involving overstatement, emotive language, and euphemism.

Overstatement

The criticism that schizophrenia is unscientific

Bentall (2003) claims that the orthodox position towards schizophrenia rests on two 'false assumptions' concerning the parsing of madness, and the role of personal psychology (Ibid., p. 8). But what he calls assumptions are in fact propositions testable by evidence. The first proposition (that madness can be divided into a small number of diseases, like schizophrenia) can be, and is, tested as criteria for mental disorders are refined. The second proposition is that a person's symptoms of madness cannot be understood in terms of the person's psychology. An orthodox biopsychosocial perspective rejects this, while some dissenters, portraying orthodox views as largely biological, accept the proposition. Again, the position can be tested according to evidence.

Bentall (2003, p. 155) first incorrectly represents propositions about schizophrenia as 'assumptions,' then overstates the position of orthodox psychiatry. He maintains that many current approaches to his assumptions are dressed in the outward appearance of being scientific. However, they 'have more in common with astrology than rational science' (Ibid.). But to equate evidential debate with astrology is misleading rhetoric, overstating the position. Orthodox psychiatry settles for looking at evidence, not evoking superstition.

Negative depiction of genetic research

In bloated language, critics depict psychiatric molecular genetic research as 'massively plagued' by false positive results. Regarding schizophrenia and other psychiatric disorders, there has been a 'stunning and unexpected *failure*' to find genes related to these conditions (Joseph, 2013, p. 84, italics in original). Uncritically accepting conclusions of schizophrenia twin and adoption researchers is 'an appalling development' in the history of scientific studies (Joseph, 2013, p. 85). Also, in genetic research, there has been disregard of 'massive flaws' (Ibid.).

Critics emphasise rigid belief and absolute certainty to the point of overstatement, in referring to researchers' work. Dissenters claim that 'psychiatric molecular genetic researchers' have tried to establish genes for schizophrenia. But their work has been based on the view that family, twin, and adoption research have demonstrated that schizophrenia is genetically based. However, this is a 'widespread but mistaken belief' (Joseph, 2013, 83). Furthermore, researchers hold as a 'belief that it is beyond question' that schizophrenia is 'highly heritable' (Ibid., p. 83). Note the term 'belief' suggesting faith rather than a hypothesis, so seeking to undermine the scientific foundations of the research.

But such research does not have to be based on a 'belief that is beyond question.' It can be guided by indications that there could be a genetic aspect to familial schizophrenia. Researchers may maintain that 'genes almost certainly play some role in the causation of schizophrenia' even though 'modest.' Contemporary researchers can recognise familial influences as well as genetic ones (Torrey, 2019, p. 133). Overstatement ignores these more nuanced positions.

Evidence that antipsychotics are implicated in brain anomalies in schizophrenia

Read (2013a) maintains that while some researchers argue against brain changes in schizophrenia implicating drugs, two recent developments 'proved otherwise' (Ibid., p. 60). So, what are these two developments?

Firstly, Dorph-Petersen et al. (2005) refer to longer-term exposure to antipsychotics in non-human primates being 'associated with' reduction in their brain volume. They observe that antipsychotics 'may confound postmortem studies and longitudinal imaging studies' of people with schizophrenia where the research depends on measures of brain volume (Ibid.).

Clearly, the study does not claim to 'prove' that drugs reduce brain volume as Read (2013a) implies.

Secondly, a longitudinal study (Ho et al., 2011) of first-episode schizophrenia concluded that their research, 'suggests that antipsychotics have a subtle but measurable influence on brain tissue loss over time' (Ibid.). Again, Read overstates the findings which do not 'prove' his view (Ibid., p. 60).

Read (2013a) cites and overstates other reviews. Weinmann and Aderhold (2011) report on evidence for frontal grey matter reduction. This '**seems to be** accelerated by antipsychotic treatment and **may** depend on cumulative doses' (Ibid., bold added). Findings from a review by Navari and Dazan (2009) '**suggest** that antipsychotics act regionally rather than globally on the brain.' Also, treatment by antipsychotics, '**potentially contributes**' to structural changes in the brain that are observed in psychosis (Ibid., bold added). Yet Read (2013a) states that these reviews 'find numerous studies confirming that antipsychotics are related to reductions in brain volume and increases in ventricles' (ibid., p. 68). But clearly, the reviews do not 'confirm' this.

The possible role of childhood trauma in schizophrenia

Torrey (2019) recognises that traumatic childhood events can leave enduring 'psychic scars,' while sexual abuse of children has been 'plausibly linked' to some mental disorders (Ibid., p. 141). Also, a few scientifically sound studies report a correlation between childhood trauma and the development of schizophrenia (e.g., Cohen, 2011).

However, Suser and Widom (2012) note that 'in almost all studies, the measure of childhood adversity is weak' and is prone to bias that might create an association with psychosis which is only an artefact of the research (Ibid., p. 672). Also, nearly all the associations reported between childhood problems and psychosis are founded on recalling childhood adversity much later. Yet, 'an extensive literature has cast doubt on the validity of retrospective reports' (Ibid.).

Read (2013a) refers to studies of identical twins where one has schizophrenia and has larger ventricles (citing Copolov and Crook, 2000, p. 109). Read (2013a) suggests that currently unidentified environmental factors may lead to increased ventricular volume, for example trauma particularly in childhood (Ibid., pp. 67–68). However, he then overreaches the evidence. He begins, 'Given that the majority of people diagnosed with 'schizophrenia' had been abused or neglected as children' before concluding that this would explain much of the supposed evidence that schizophrenia is a disease of the brain (Ibid., pp. 67–68).

But Read (2013a) does not cite research showing that 'the majority' of people with schizophrenia have been abused or neglected. It is unclear how 'abuse' and 'neglect' are being defined. It is not evident if the reported accounts are retrospective, or how reliable they are. Such issues are evaded in the phrase, 'Given that' making the claims overstated.

Faustian allusions to sedating side effects of antipsychotics

Davies (2014) accepts that using antipsychotics leads to the intensity of psychotic symptoms being reduced. Antipsychotics also, as he points out, have a sedating effect which he expresses as that they, 'diminish other physical, emotional functions integral to all our mental activity.'

But picking up a quote from a patient who disliked the effect of antipsychotics, Davies observes, 'It is of course up to the individual patient to decide whether paying with one's soul is an acceptable price to pay for the mitigation of their symptoms' (Ibid., pp. 288–289). How such Faustian allusions of paying with one's soul carries forward debate is unclear. It may be good rhetoric but makes a weak argument as overstatement.

Emotive language

The criticism that schizophrenia was invented

Concerning the categorisation of schizophrenia, is the claim that the disorder was 'invented.' This and characterising early developments in psychiatry as a crisis which it survived has attracted emotive rhetoric. It has been described in terms of an 'appalling cost' with people like animals 'branded' with a 'socially devastating' label (Read, 2013a, p. 32).

Criticism of a medical view of schizophrenia

Read, Mosher and Bentall (2013) arguing that schizophrenia is not an illness (Ibid., pp. 3–8) use metaphor and simile drawing on incarceration, explosives, the notion of imperialism linked with occupying forces, and hatred. Hospitals are 'dehumanising prison-like' places (Ibid., p. 4). Life events become 'triggers of an underlying genetic timebomb' (Ibid.). Dominance of a biological view reflects '… a colonisation of the psychological and social by the biological' which has involved the 'vilification' of studies that indicated the role of contextual factors in causing schizophrenia (Ibid.). Such exaggerated and emotive language is unconvincing and lacking in argument.

Criticisms of the efficacy of ECT

Petrides and Braga (2009) describe pioneering work by Ugo Cerletti and Lucio Bini in straightforward terms specifying that the first patient recovered (Ibid., p. 290). Read, Mosher and Bentall (2013) present a dissenting view of the same events. They state that Cerletti experimented with dogs, placing electrodes in their 'mouth and rectum' and that 'many died.' His notion of using electrodes occurred to Cerletti in 'a slaughterhouse.'

There he witnessed 'hogs electrocuted.' He 'found' his first patients who was 'a homeless man at a railway station' (Ibid., p. 90).

The second account is coloured and emotive to convey distaste of the procedure. But why is placing electrodes in the mouth and rectum of dogs and that many died relevant to the effectiveness of ECT with people? Why mention a 'slaughterhouse' and 'hogs' unless to suggest that Cerletti devalued human life? When Cerletti 'found' his first patient, was he scouring railway stations for homeless people to experiment on? The message is, if this was the foundation of ECT, contemporary practitioners cannot value human life. Crucially, the account ignores that the patient recovered. Rhetoric has replaced argument.

ECT and 'brain damage'

Read, Mosher and Bentall (2013) say that in the past (1940s and 1950s) autopsies indicated evidence of brain damage, 'including necrosis' (Ibid., p. 96). UK ECT Review Group, 2003) found ECT an effective short-term treatment for depression but state that after ECT the use of CT scans, 'confirmed frontal lobe atrophy' (Read, Mosher and Bentall, 2013, p. 96). Also, an MRI study found that the number of ECT treatments administered was 'correlated with reduced grey matter density' (citing Shah et al., 2002). Furthermore, in several regions of the cortex, has been found 'marked deactivation' (citing Schmidt et al., 2008).

Davies (2014) observes that, many psychiatrists 'still swear by the healing effects' of ECT.

But their 'claims' about success are greatly overtaken by 'reams of research' which shows for ECT, 'widespread neurological damage' (Ibid.). Note that psychiatrists 'swear' by healing effects as if unflinchingly committed and bound by their views. 'Reams' of research are mentioned as if quantity were decisive over quality.

However, NICE (2003, 2009, 2014) guidance states that the mortality with ECT does not exceed 'that associated with the administration of a general anaesthetic for minor surgery' (section 3.4). Also, six reviewed studies provided no evidence that ECT causes brain damage (NICE, 2003, 2009, 2014, section 4.1.8).

Euphemism

The criticism that schizophrenia was invented

Claims (e.g., Read, 2013a, p. 20) that schizophrenia was 'invented' as a piece of fantasy by psychiatry pioneers Kraepelin and Bleuler are unsubstantiated. Representing the invention of schizophrenia as a continuing search for categories of 'unusual behaviours' is euphemistic. Euphemising disturbing and potentially harmful behaviour associated with schizophrenia as simply 'unusual behaviours' allows critics to castigate those who see it as an illness.

Weaknesses of proposing continua as an alternative to categorisation

Critics of categorisation may propose a continuum which joins together disorder and wellness so that 'no clear dividing line is recognised between "psychosis" and other thoughts, feelings and beliefs' (Cooke, 2017, p. 6, Executive Summary). But symptoms of psychosis are generally so different in degree to what most people experience that they effectively become different in kind.

Some people may hear voices to a minor or intense degree. But to say that given enough stress, such experiences may 'shade into psychosis' (Cooke, 2017, p. 113, section 14.1) suggests a spurious closeness between ordinarily hearing voices and psychosis. Thought disorder in psychosis may be equated with getting mixed up when we are 'emotionally stressed,' yet in psychiatric guidance it involves disorganisation 'so severe as to substantially impair communication' (American Psychiatric Association, 2013, p. 107). Delusions might be likened to having strong beliefs that 'others around you do not share' (Cooke, 2017, p. 10, section 1.1) but in diagnostic guidance 'fixed beliefs that are not amenable to change in the light of conflicting evidence' (American Psychiatric Association, 2013, p. 107).

Other rhetoric

Laudatory presentation of supportive evidence

Contrasting to critics' mistrustful presentation of evidence concerning drug companies, an MRI study associating antipsychotic drugs and brain volume (Ho et al., 2011) has been conveyed in laudatory terms. Emphasising perceived strengths of the research Read (2013a) says that the study involved '674 brain scans, on 211 patients (**far more than most previous studies**).' It lasted on average for '7.2 years (**the longest to date**).' (Ibid., p. 69, bold added).

He describes the publication in which the article appeared as the '**most prestigious psychiatry journal**.' The findings were announced to the press in September 2008 by Nancy Andreasen the '**esteemed neuroscientist**' who is '**famous** for her separation of positive and negative symptoms' (Ibid., bold added). Prestige, esteem, and fame as appeals to authority are irrelevant to arguments that the research is convincing or otherwise.

Critics misrepresenting an orthodox position about antipsychotics

Contrary to rhetoric used by Davies (2014), an orthodox position does not claim that antibiotics cure ('fix') schizophrenia, but rather that the drugs reduce certain symptoms. Neither is it held that antipsychotics rebalance brain chemicals to an optimum level. The dopamine hypotheses for example have evolved into more precise understandings.

So, for Davies to say that there exists no research which confirms that antipsychotics 'fix any known brain abnormality,' or that there is no evidence that they '"rebalance" brain chemistry to some optimum level' is irrelevant to current debates (Davies, 2014, p. 288). Similarly, he states of antipsychotics that 'inflated claims about their ability to "cure" mental disorder are [as] unsubstantiated' (Ibid., p. 287). Here it is obvious that antipsychotics do not offer a cure. Also, inflated claims about anything are (by definition) unsubstantiated.

Conflicting/weak evidence

As well as using rhetorical devices, criticisms of schizophrenia refer to conflicting or weak evidence.

Weaknesses of using symptoms for identification and assessment instead of categorisation

Some critics, rejecting categorisation, propose focusing on symptoms of schizophrenia like hallucinations. Independently analysed hallucination and delusion severity scores are associated with different patterns of neuropsychological functioning (Cohen and Docherty, 2005). However, problems of reliability arose with symptoms (Mojtabai and Rieder, 1998). Bentall (2013, pp. 144–145) argues that some reported measures of reliability of symptoms may underestimate what can be achieved by specially designed assessments.

Criticisms that the 'medical model' is pessimistic

Some dissenters claim that what they call the medical model of schizophrenia had led to 'unwarranted and destructive pessimism' about the likelihood of recovery (Read, Mosher and Bentall, 2013, p. 3). Campbell (2010) says that the medical model encouraged his view of 'having a chronic and incurable illness' (Ibid., p. 22). Edwards (quoted in Cooke, 2017) speaks of a self-help group assisting her to reject that she was 'a psychiatric patient with a lifelong brain disease' (Ibid., section 9.2.1).

However, this pessimistic view about recovery is itself overly pessimistic. Various studies of long-term follow-up and prognosis for schizophrenia show a quite different picture (e.g., Harding et al., 1987; Lieberman et al., 1993). Reviewing these findings, Torrey (2019) notes that for schizophrenia, for an average patient, the 30-year course is more favourable than the ten-year course. This contradicts 'a widespread stereotype of the disease' which can be traced to Kraepelin's view that 'most patients slowly deteriorate' (Ibid., p. 101).

Proposing that understanding schizophrenia as an illness is just another theory

The report *Understanding Psychosis and Schizophrenia* (Cooke, 2017) proposes that a medical perspective is merely one of many views each of which might carry equal or greater weight. It says that referring to hearing voices as symptoms of mental disorder, or schizophrenia, or psychosis is 'only one way of thinking about them' (Cooke, 2017, p. 6, Executive Summary). Thinking of hearing voices as symptoms of illness perhaps caused by a 'problem in the brain,' is 'just one of the theories' (Ibid., p. 17, section 3, Introduction).

Yet such a claim underplays the role of evidence from observation or research that one view is more accurate (or more in line with the evidence) than another. Instead, one is invited to accept that everyone might have a different view and no one person's view is any better than another's. This avoids judgement and evaluation about what is said.

Biogenetic causal beliefs involve negative attitudes, and psychosocial beliefs positive attitudes

Read, Haslam and Magliano (2013) represent 'mental health literacy' as attempting to destigmatise schizophrenia for the public, by emphasising it is an illness, like any other physical ailment. This could effectively publicise schizophrenia's psychiatric background and biological basis, and its treatment including by medication. They itemise 22 correlational studies reporting associations between causal beliefs, whether biogenetic or psychosocial, and attitudes (from sematic differential choices) or desire for social distance (from behavioural intention questionnaires). They note 17 experimental studies for example showing a video of the same person but with different causal explanations to two different groups of respondents. These studies strongly associated biogenetic causal beliefs with negative attitudes, and psychosocial beliefs with positive attitudes (Ibid., pp. 160–166).

However, 16 of the 22 correlational studies, and only 5 of the 17 experiments concerned schizophrenia specifically. Weakening findings further, all studies concerned projected attitudes not real-world behaviour. Also, studies giving volunteers a choice of mental disorder owing to biological causes or psychosocial ones polarise the causal factors. A more rounded causal picture (e.g., National Library of Medicine, 2021) would implicate biological, psychological, and social influences.

Mistrustful presentation of evidence from research involving drug companies

Critics may question research on brain anomalies in schizophrenia, simply by citing drug company involvement without reference to the quality of the studies. It is claimed that reviews find that 'numerous studies' confirm that antipsychotic medication is related to reduced brain volume and increased brain ventricles. Also, 'industry-sponsored studies' tried to prove that such findings applied to first-generation antipsychotic drugs, but not newer atypical ones (Read, 2013a, p. 60).

Claims that those with schizophrenia in developing countries do better with less access to antipsychotics

Press coverage (e.g., Whitaker, 2010) sometimes suggests that in developing countries schizophrenia has a better outcome than in high income countries, including when not treated with antipsychotics. In a review, Cohen et al. (2008) argue that evidence presents 'a far more complex picture' and that we should re-examine the projected outcome of schizophrenia in low- and middle-income countries (Ibid., Conclusions). Jablensky and Sartorius (2008) challenge Cohen et al. (2008) representation of the World Health Organisation data to which their observations largely referred.

However, Sullivan, Allen and Nero (2007) studying Palau in the western Pacific note that the republic has 'one of the highest rates of schizophrenia in the world today.' They challenge the assumption from cross-cultural research that schizophrenia in 'necessarily more benign in "developing" countries' (Ibid., p. 189). Alem and colleagues (2009) looking at rural Ethiopia note the very small proportion of participants experiencing complete remission. They state that this supports the view in developing countries, schizophrenia outcome may be 'heterogeneous rather than uniformly favourable' (Ibid., p. 654).

Referring to an editorial by Lewis (2011) on antipsychotic medication and brain volume, Read (2013a) disparagingly mentions that it was written by someone 'who discloses income from eight drug companies' (Ibid., p. 69). The editorial mentions the benefits of reductions in cortical grey matter made in adolescence being accompanied by improvements in cognitive capacity. Read (2013a) cites researchers who sarcastically suggest that Lewis is effectively saying that patients with psychosis may have 'too much brain in the first place.' These critics are approvingly said to be 'of a less ideological bent.' Also, they have 'no drug company sponsorship' (Ibid., p. 69).

Read (2013a) cites the findings of a paper jointly authored by Ho et al. (2011) and reported, attributed to Andreasen, in the press three years before the paper was published (*New York Times*, 2008). This seemingly means that 'Biological psychiatry' and the 'pharmaceutical industry' had three years to get ready their response to this 'proof' that antipsychotics rather than the mental disorder was causing the 'brain atrophy' (Read, 2013a, p. 69). Is Read really maintaining that someone purposely allowed drug companies plenty of time to prepare a response? Overstatement and innuendo begins to muddy the waters. Also, the vague terms 'biological psychiatry' and 'the pharmaceutical industry' in not identifying individuals, prevents such individuals from challenging what is said.

References

Alem, A., Kebede, D., Fekadu, A., Shibre, T., Fekadu, D., Beyero, T., Medhin, G., Negash, A. and Kullgren, G. (2009) 'Clinical course and outcome of schizophrenia in a predominantly treatment-naïve cohort in rural Ethiopia' *Schizophrenia Bulletin* 35, 646–654. https://www.ncbi.nlm.nih.gov/pmc/articles/PMC2669573/

American Psychiatric Association (2013) *Diagnostic and Statistical Manual of Mental Disorders Fifth Edition (DSM5)*. Washington DC, APA.

Bentall, R. (2003) *Madness Explained: Psychosis and Human Nature*. London, Penguin Books.

Campbell, P. (2010) 'Surviving the system' in Bassett, T. and Stickley, T. (Eds.) *Voices of Experience*. Chichester, Wiley-Blackwell (p. 22).

Cohen, A., Patel, V., Thara, R. and Gureje, O. (2008) 'Questioning an axiom: Better prognosis for schizophrenia in the developing world?' *Schizophrenia Bulletin* 34, 229–244. https://www.ncbi.nlm.nih.gov/pmc/articles/PMC2632419/

Cohen, A. S. and Docherty, N. M. (2005) 'Symptom orientated versus syndrome approaches to resolving heterogeneity of neuropsychological functioning in schizophrenia' *Neuropsychiatry* 17, 3, 384–390. https://neuro.psychiatryonline.org/doi/10.1176/jnp.17.3.384

Cohen, P. (2011) 'Abuse in childhood and the risk for psychotic symptoms in later life' *American Journal of Psychiatry* 2011, 168, 7–8. https://ajp.psychiatryonline.org/doi/full/10.1176/appi.ajp.2010.10101513

Cooke, A. (Ed.) (2017) *Understanding Psychosis and Schizophrenia: Why People Sometimes Hear Voices, Believe Things that Others Find Strange, or Appear*

Out of Touch with Reality, and What Can Help. Canterbury, British Psychological Society Division of Clinical Psychology/ Canterbury Christchurch University.

Copolov, D. and Crook, J. (2000) 'Biological markers and schizophrenia' *Australian and New Zealand Journal of Psychiatry* 34, S108–S112.

Davies, J. (2014) *Cracked: Why Psychiatry Is Doing More Harm than Good.* London, Icon Books.

Dorph-Petersen, K.-A., Pierri, J. N., Perel, J. M., Zhuoxin, S., Sampson, A. R. and Lewis, D. A. (2005) 'The influence of chronic exposure to antipsychotic medications on brain size before and after tissue fixation: A comparison of haloperidol and olanzapine in macaque monkeys' *Neuropsychopharmacology* 30, 9, 1649–1661 (September). www.semanticscholar.org/paper/The-Influence-of-Chronic-Exposure-to-Antipsychotic-Dorph%E2%80%90Petersen-Pierri/f2f4af5c5a2c394266c37b9dd898ba1688607ad0

Goldacre (2012) *Bad Pharma: How Drug Companies Mislead Doctors and Harm Patients.* London, Fourth Estate.

Harding, C. M., Brooks, G. W., Ashikaga, T., Strauss, J. S. and Breier, A. (1987) 'The Vermont longitudinal study of persons with severe mental illness, I: Methodology, study sample, and overall status 32 years later' *American Journal of Psychiatry* 144, 6, 718–725 (June). https://pubmed.ncbi.nlm.nih.gov/3591991/

Ho, B.-C., Andreasen, N., Ziebell, S., Pierson, R. and Magnotta, V. (2011) 'Long-term antipsychotic treatment and brain volumes: A longitudinal study of first-episode schizophrenia' *Archives of General Psychiatry* 68, 2, 128–137. https://pubmed.ncbi.nlm.nih.gov/21300943/

Jablensky, A. and Sartorius, N. (2008) 'What did the WHO studies really find?' *Schizophrenia Bulletin* 34, 2, 253–255. https://www.semanticscholar.org/paper/What-Did-the-WHO-Studies-Really-Find-Jablensky-Sartorius/c375847ae99e0b5519bc0a35ba4b2a6ccba3ca38

Joseph, J. (2013) '"Schizophrenia" and heredity: Why the emperor (still) has no genes' in Read, J. and Dillon, J. (Eds.) (2nd Edition) *Models of Madness: Psychological, Social and Biological Approaches to Psychosis.* London and New York, Routledge (pp. 72–89).

Lewis, D. (2011) 'Antipsychotic medication and brain volume' *Archives of General Psychiatry* 68, 126–127.

Lieberman, J., Jody, D., Geisler, S., Alvir, J., Loebel, A., Szymanski, S., Woerner, M. and Borenstein, M. (1993) 'Time course and biologic correlates of treatment response in first-episode schizophrenia' *Archives of General Psychiatry* 50, 369–376. https://pubmed.ncbi.nlm.nih.gov/8098203/

Mojtabai, R. and Rieder, R. O. (1998) 'Limitations of the symptom-orientated approach to psychiatric research' *British Journal of Psychiatry* 173, 198–202.

National Library of Medicine (2021) 'What does it mean to have a genetic predisposition to a disease?' *National Library of Medicine*, Bethesda, Maryland (May 2021). https://medlineplus.gov/genetics/understanding/mutationsanddisorders/predisposition/

Navari, S. and Dazan, P. (2009) 'Do antipsychotic drugs affect brain structure? A systematic and critical review of MRI findings' *Psychological Medicine* 39, 1363–1377. https://pubmed.ncbi.nlm.nih.gov/19338710/

NICE (2003, 2009, 2014) *Guidance on the use of electroconvulsive therapy: Technology appraisal guidance TA 59* (Published 2003, Updated 2009, Static list review 2014). www.nice.org.uk/guidance/ta59

Petrides, G. and Braga, R. J. (2009) 'Electroconvulsive therapy in schizophrenia' in Kasper, S. and Papadimitriou, G. N. (Eds.) (2nd Edition) *Schizophrenia: Biopsychosocial Approaches and Current Challenges* (Medical Psychiatry Series). New York and London, Informa Healthcare (pp. 290–298).

Read, J. (2013a) 'Biological psychiatry's lost cause: The schizophrenic brain' in Read, J. and Dillon, J. (Eds.) (2nd Edition) *Models of Madness: Psychological, Social and Biological Approaches to Psychosis.* London and New York, Routledge (pp. 62–71).

Read, J., Haslam, N. and Magliano, L. (2013) 'Prejudice, stigma and 'schizophrenia': The role of bio-genetic ideology' in Read, J. and Dillon, J. (Eds.) (2nd Edition) *Models of Madness: Psychological, Social and Biological Approaches to Psychosis.* London and New York, Routledge (pp. 157–177).

Read, J., Mosher, L. and Bentall, R. (2013) 'Schizophrenia is not an illness' in Read, J. and Dillon, J. (Eds.) (2nd Edition) *Models of Madness: Psychological, Social and Biological Approaches to Psychosis.* London and New York, Routledge (pp. 3–8).

Schmidt, E., Reininghaus, B., Enzinger, C., Ebner, C., Hoffmann, P. and Kapfhammer, P. (2008) 'Changes in brain metabolism after ECT' *Journal of Affective Disorders* 106, 203–208.

Shah, P. J., Glabus, M. F., Goodwin, G. M. and Ebmeier, K. P. (2002) 'Chronic treatment-resistant depression and right fronto-spatial atrophy' *British Journal of Psychiatry* 180, 434–440.

Sullivan, R. J., Allen, J. S. and Nero, K. L. (2007) 'Schizophrenia in Palau: A biocultural analysis' *Current Anthropology* 48, 189–213. https://www.semanticscholar.org/paper/Schizophrenia-in-Palau-Sullivan-Allen/223ecf7cd81d759e06ff4fddcdcd5322a9e09584

Suser, E. and Widom, C. S. (2012) 'Still searching for lost truths about the bitter sorrows of childhood' *Schizophrenia Bulletin* 38, 4, 672–675 (18 June). https://academic.oup.com/schizophreniabulletin/article/38/4/672/1871240

The UK ECT Review Group (2003) 'Efficacy and safety of ECT in depressive disorders' *Lancet* 361, 799–808.

Torrey, E. F. (2019) (7th edition) *Surviving Schizophrenia: A Family Manual.* New York and London, Harper Perennial.

Weinmann, S. and Aderhold, V. (2011) 'Antipsychotic medication, mortality and neurodegeneration' *Psychosis* 2, 50–69. https://www.researchgate.net/publication/233138682_Antipsychotic_medication_mortality_and_neurodegeneration_The_need_for_more_selective_use_and_lower_doses

Whitaker, R. (2010) *Anatomy of an Epidemic: Magic Bullets, Psychiatric Drugs, and the Astonishing Rise of Mental Illness in America.* New York, Crown.

12

FURTHER CRITICISMS

Introduction

Following on from the previous chapter, this one examines further criticisms of research into schizophrenia and understanding of the disorder. I point out the weaknesses of these criticisms. Regarding distorting emphases, the chapter considers disputable slants when reviewing genetic research. I examine criticism putting the spotlight on side effects of antipsychotics rather on reducing or avoiding any such adverse consequences. Also discussed are dissenters' views of ECT-related deaths which may place a misleading emphasis on older research, and critics laying stress on the simplistic, outdated, reductionist, unsubstantiated, contextless, and crude.

Turning to illogical criticisms and positions, I look at criticisms that physical causes demand physical treatments for schizophrenia, and dissenters proposing subjectivism over medical evidence.

Misrepresenting biopsychosocial psychiatry as purely biological is reviewed. I examine the criticism that stigma towards schizophrenia stems from 'biological psychiatry,' and the misrepresentation that orthodox researchers envisage a purely chemical 'solution' to schizophrenia. I also look at the dissenting view that 'failed' neurochemical explanations undermine justifications for using antipsychotics.

In considering focusing on old research or old versions of a theory or explanation, the chapter reviews the criticism that original dopamine hypothesis is still current and 'popular' and is simplistic and unsubstantiated. As well, I consider the criticism that researchers have continually failed

DOI: 10.4324/9781003413554-12

to confirm the dopamine ('lead') hypothesis, the citing of earlier negative studies of ECT efficacy, and critics' potentially misleading reference to old ECT research.

Under the umbrella of a redefinition of torture, I discuss the distortion that coercive treatment may and medically indicated involuntary treatment may each constitute torture, and that the doctrine of medical necessity hinders protection from abuses. Also, the chapter considers the criticism that solitary confinement and restraint may constitute torture, that guardianship should not allow justification of forced treatment, the view that institutionalising legislation should be abolished, and the criticism that severity of mental illness should not justify deprivation of liberty.

Finally, under 'other criticisms' I examine dissenting views referring misleadingly to a genetic 'basis' of schizophrenia, criticising of nebulous targets, and imputed (sometimes malign) motivations in genetic research. The chapter looks at the view that only after the dopamine hypothesis had failed researchers considered other neurochemicals, and the issue of ECT historical cases being conflated with modern findings.

Distorting emphases

Disputable emphases reviewing genetic research

Family, twin, and adoption studies constitutes early pre-molecular research into heritability and schizophrenia. Cardno and Gottesman (2000) cite earlier research on schizophrenia from 1963 to 1987 showing higher rates for MZ (48%) than for DZ twins (17%). A meta-analysis of twin studies estimated the genetic liability to schizophrenia at 81% (Sullivan, Kendler and Neale, 2003).

However, contemporary researchers reject high estimates of heritability of schizophrenia of 80% or more (Torrey, 2019, p. 132). Indeed, it is observed that, 'classical twin design remains controversial' (Henriksen, Nordgaard and Jansson, 2017, pp. 4–5). Accordingly, Schosser and McGuffin (2009) in a book chapter on genetics and schizophrenia devote one page to family and twin studies and four to recent genetic research including GWAS (Ibid., p. 84).

Yet some dissenters still emphasise the old, indirect genetic deductions. In a chapter on genetics, Joseph (2013) covers 11 printed pages with reports of family, twin, and adoption studies, and only two on contemporary research for genes relating to schizophrenia. More recently, Joseph (2023) takes a similar view. Focusing on older genetic deductions rather than recent studies can be misleading.

Criticism emphasising adverse effects of antipsychotics rather how to reduce or avoid these effects

Orthodox practitioners accept that antipsychotics can cause unpleasant side effects. However, they may differ from dissenters in recognising the choices that are available among different antipsychotic medications, and practical steps that can be taken to mitigate adverse effects.

In their chapter, 'Antipsychotic drugs' Hutton et al. (2013) discuss, what they consider to be increasing evidence that antipsychotic medication contributes to mortality. Looking at weight gain, they mention levels of risk of different drugs ranging from 30% to 7%. However, overlooking implications for a patient and clinician choosing an antipsychotic with lowest risk, they state, 'This situation is concerning because metabolic syndrome doubles the 10-year risk of coronary heart disease' (Ibid., pp. 110–116).

By contrast, Torrey (2019) discusses practicalities of choosing specific antipsychotics to mitigate side effects. For example, regarding sedation, he cites antipsychotics that are least likely to cause it namely 'aripiprazole (Abilify), iloperidone (Fanapt) or paliperidone (Invega)' (Ibid., p. 180).

ECT-related deaths – misleading emphasis on older research

Read, Mosher and Bentall (2013, pp. 97–99) select studies 'finding significantly higher ECT-related death rates than official statements' including a 1980 Scotland study with a death rate of 1/92. (Ibid., table 8.1, p. 98). They conclude that many findings depend on those who administer the ECT treatment reporting the deaths. What they believe was a more objective measure was 'accidentally provided' by a study of patients' attitudes by Freeman and Kendall (1980) who proposed to interview 183 people a year after they had received ECT. This old research found that 12 patients had died, four having 'killed themselves.' Read, Mosher and Bentall (2013) note that if one counts only the two deaths that happened during ECT treatment, the 'death rate was one per 91.5' (Ibid., p. 99).

How does this supposedly more objective past measure compare with recent reviews of evidence? NICE (2003, 2009, 2014) found no evidence to suggest that 'the mortality associated with ECT is greater than that associated with minor procedures involving general anaesthetics' (Ibid., section 4.1.8).

Emphasising the simplistic, outdated, reductionist, unsubstantiated, contextless, and crude

Cooke (2017) castigates reliance on a 'simplistic' medical model (Ibid., section 13.1). Edwards (in Cooke, 2017) speaks of an 'outdated' medical model (Ibid., section 9.2.1). Read, Mosher and Bentall (2013) mention

'Simplistic and reductionist' genetic and biological theories leading to 'lobotomising, electroshocking or drugging of millions of people.' We should eschew such 'unsubstantiated' approaches. Some medical professionals seem to accept that human experience can be boiled down to 'a single, contextless, medical sounding word.' They try to explain madness with the 'crude' ideas and approaches of 'biological psychiatry' (Ibid., pp. 3–5).

But if mental health professionals adhere to models and approaches that are simplistic, outdated, reductionist, unsubstantiated, contextless, and crude, this is (by definition) pointless. As a rhetorical device, narrowing criticism to a model or approach that is self-evidently weak, blunts the point.

Illogical criticisms and positions

Criticisms that physical causes demand physical treatments for schizophrenia

Seeing schizophrenia as a physical illness, dissenters may claim, assumes that it demands solely physical treatment like medication, or ECT (Read, Mosher and Bentall, 2013, pp. 4–5). Campbell (2010) sees a medical model as encouraging 'a resort to exclusively physical treatments' (Ibid.).

However, such claims are illogical and unsupported by evidence. Physical causes form only part of the picture. Information from the National Health Service in England (NHS, reviewed 2019) indicates that in schizophrenia, 'a combination of physical, genetic, psychological and environmental factors' are influential in whether someone develops the disorder. Also, a psychotic episode could be brought about by, 'a stressful or emotional life event' (Ibid.). Furthermore, nonphysical treatments form a part of orthodox approaches. Torrey (2019, p. 198) taking a medical perspective of schizophrenia, discusses herbal treatments, cognitive-behavioural therapy, and family therapy (Ibid., p. 201). Similarly, Granholm and Loh (2009, pp. 270–274) envisage a range of recommended provision from family interventions to supported employment (Ibid.).

Proposing subjectivism over medical evidence

Subjectivism proposes that knowledge is subjective and personal and that there is no external or objective truth because different people differ in beliefs and perceptions about knowledge. So, what is true for one person may not be so for another. Subjectivism eschews examining whether a position is true or correct. In discussing schizophrenia, importance is attached to what 'some people' think or feel as though personal and subjective views and experiences imply agreed objective truth.

Cooke (2017) suggests that what is important is not so much whether schizophrenia (or psychosis) is an illness according to medical evidence. Rather, it is whether people 'think of themselves' as having an illness (Ibid., p. 6, Executive Summary); or whether they 'find it helpful to think of their problems as an illness' (Ibid., p. 103).

The difficulty with this is that if the statement 'truth is subjective' is taken as an unconditional claim, it is self-refuting. If the statement is interpreted subjectively, it lacks significance (Baghramian, 2001, abstract).

Misrepresenting biopsychosocial psychiatry as purely biological

The criticism that stigma towards schizophrenia stems from 'biological psychiatry'

Regarding stigma, dissenters identify supposed negative effects of a predominantly biological view of schizophrenia which they equate with orthodox biopsychosocial psychiatry. For dissenters, drug companies promote a view of schizophrenia as an illness, leading to more use of drugs and greater discrimination. Drug company websites untrustworthily portray schizophrenia as a 'debilitating disease' and a biologically based illness (Read, Haslam and Magliano, 2013, p. 160). It is said, spending large sums of money, predominantly from pharmaceutical firms, to 'teach the public to think like biological psychiatrists' has led to greater discrimination and the greater use of medication (Ibid., p. 165).

Read, Haslam and Magliano (2013) in discussing prejudice, stigma and schizophrenia refer to the role of 'bio-genetic ideology.' This overlooks that, where research in biopsychosocial psychiatry examines factors like genetics, it will naturally focus on physical and biological aspects. However, genetics also forms part of a wider framework. Critics mislead in presenting biological aspects of psychiatry as isolated from psychological and social aspects and equating orthodox biopsychosocial psychiatry with this caricature of biological psychiatry.

The criticism that orthodox researchers envisage a purely chemical response to schizophrenia

Read (2013a) states that the majority of researchers of schizophrenia persist in seeking a 'purely bio-chemical solution.' Recently this has implicated glutamate and other neurochemicals. Others researchers 'more productively' seek to link biochemistry to psychological and social factors (Ibid., p. 66). This view overlooks that researchers examining the influence of neurochemicals will focus on these, but not precluding awareness of psychological and environmental factors.

Howes and Kapur (2009) reviewed evidence including environmental risk factors hypothesising that environmental stress and substance abuse interact with a genetic susceptibility, leading to dopamine dysregulation. Selten and Cantor-Graae (2005) propose that long-term experience of social defeat (SD) – negative experience of being excluded from the majority group – may increase risk of schizophrenia. Selten et al. (2013) found that evidence for SD increasing risk of schizophrenia was strongest for migration and childhood trauma. They argue that SD gives a 'parsimonious and plausible' explanation for several epidemiological findings that are unexplainable solely by 'genetic confounding' (Ibid.).

The criticism that 'failed' neurochemical explanations undermine justifications for using antipsychotics

Critics may say that the dopamine theory has become 'the cornerstone' of claims that schizophrenia is an illness (Read, 2013a, p. 66). Commentators focusing on confirmation of the original dopamine theory having 'failed' can imply that schizophrenia is not an illness with neurochemical features. Consequently, the use of medication with a presumed action relating to dopamine dysregulation is unjustified. This would contradict the marketing of pharmaceutical companies basing drug promotion solely on a claimed effect on the earlier proposed simple dopamine dysregulation.

However, the evolving dopamine hypothesis modified according to new evidence, is argued to be conversant with the use of medication which includes action on the dopamine system. For example, Jauhar and colleagues (2017) state that their findings concerning dopamine in schizophrenia was consistent with a transdiagnostic role for dopamine dysfunction in the development of psychosis. They note that this suggests dopamine synthesis capacity as a potential novel drug target for schizophrenia (and bipolar disorder).

Focusing on old research or old versions of a theory or explanation

The criticism that the original dopamine hypothesis is still current and 'popular'

Critics have stated that 'Biological psychiatry's lead theory of schizophrenia, for the past 40 years, is that it is caused by too much dopamine' (Read, 2013a, p. 64). However, the present tense in this expression misleads. The 'too much dopamine' hypothesis was the original version of a theory reflecting evidence available at the time.

The hypothesis evolved according to new evidence and in relation to new technology and procedures (Howes and Kapur, 2009). However, critics maintain that the early theory remains 'very popular' (Read, 2013a, p. 64) but whatever, 'very popular' might mean in this context, this surely cannot apply to the researchers who developed later versions or others aware of later refinements.

The criticism that original dopamine theory is simplistic and unsubstantiated

Read (2013a) refers to 'the original, simplistic, and unsubstantiated dopamine theory' (Ibid., p. 66). Anything 'simplistic' rather than 'simple' in the positive sense is unlikely to be useful, making the description of the early theory as 'simple' a rejection of it. Also, it is true that the early theory was later found to be 'unsubstantiated' as new evidence emerged. But this is surely a strength showing that, as a scientific hypothesis, it can be rejected or, as with the dopamine hypothesis, further developed and refined.

The criticism that researchers have continually failed to confirm the dopamine ('lead') hypothesis

To speak of the 'continued failure to confirm biological psychiatry's lead hypothesis' (Read, 2013a, p. 66) is to misrepresent the nature of hypotheses in general and the dopamine hypotheses particularly. Good hypotheses are by their nature amenable to being confirmed (always provisionally) or disconfirmed. They can also be confirmed in certain aspects and not in others, leading to refinements.

Critics' citing of earlier negative studies of ECT efficacy

Read et al. (2013, p. 292) cite predominantly old studies comparing real and fake ECT showing little or no sustained difference. For example, Taylor and Fleminger (1980) found both groups improved equally. In the Leicester ECT trial (Brandon et al., 1985) both groups improved, but after six weeks the fake group performed better on all four measures used. Such studies preceded the later evolution of diagnostic criteria (*DSMIII* and later versions) and better research methodology.

Researchers advise viewing the conclusions 'with caution.' Such studies had, 'significant methodological flaws.' Having samples of 30 or less they may have lacked the power to detect differences. Most used few ECT sessions to ethically avoid giving patients prolonged sham ECT. Where patients participated at various stages of their illness and research included those with schizophreniform disorder and patients free of medication, it was problematic. Many were particularly responsive to medication which could artificially inflate the response rate in both groups (Petrides and Braga, 2009, pp. 291–292).

Critics potentially misleading citation of old ECT research

Given that interpretation of old studies on ECT requires caution, the dates of cited research must be clear. The *Hamilton Depression Rating Scale (HAM-D)* (Hamilton, 1960), a 17-item instrument completed by a clinician, measures frequency and intensity of depressive symptoms in individuals with major depressive disorder. Referring to *HAM-D*, Davies (2014) observes that 'recent reviews of ECT research' have failed to demonstrate significant differences between real and fake ECT following the procedure. Research assessing comparative improvement rates after six months revealed a two-point difference in favour of the fake treatment suggesting that any positive ECT effects are 'largely placebo' (Davies, 2014, pp. 211–212, citing Bracken et al., 2012).

Davies (2014) having referred to 'recent reviews' cites Bracken et al., 2012. In fact, this source is an article critical of some approaches in psychiatry that mentions the research in question, the Northwick Park ECT trial, of 1980 (Johnstone et al., 1980). Davies source citing could misleadingly imply that the evidence is recent.

Distorted redefinition of torture

The distortion that coercive treatment may constitute torture

A *Special Rapporteur on Torture and Other Cruel, Inhuman or Degrading Treatment or Punishment* was written by Méndez (2013). It argues that Article 12 of the *UN Convention on the Rights of Persons with Disabilities* recognises that all persons enjoy 'legal capacity' in all aspects of life on an 'equal basis with others.' Contrary to 'medical necessity' and 'best interest' doctrines, this relates coercive treatment to torture, demanding its abolition. Méndez (2013) recommends that laws or policies concerning 'substituted' decision making be replaced with 'supported' decision making. This challenges the centrality of impaired capacity to decisions made against a patient's will.

Against this, psychiatrist Paul Appelbaum states that, in Méndez' report, there is much 'slippery language.' All the report's recommendations follow from its redefinition of torture to include 'involuntary hospitalisation or treatment when people have been found incompetent to make decisions or are dangerous to self or others' (Levin, 2014).

The criticism that medically indicated involuntary treatment may constitute torture

Méndez (2013, paragraph 32) notes the discriminatory character of 'forced psychiatric interventions' including 'non-consensual medication' involving people with psychosocial disabilities. This, he maintains, satisfies intent and purpose required under Article 1 of the Convention against Torture, despite claims of good intentions by medical professionals.

Lieberman, Levin and Ruiz (2013) maintain that medically indicated involuntary treatment used in appropriate circumstances 'can restore the functional and decisional capacity' of people having severe psychiatric disorders. This protects the person and others from 'the behavioural consequences of their conditions.'

The criticism that the doctrine of medical necessity hinders protection from abuses

Méndez (2013, paragraph 35) maintains that the notion of medical necessity, gets in the way of protection from 'arbitrary abuses in health-care settings.' Therefore, treatment that violates the Convention on the Rights of Persons with Disabilities, whether involving coercion or discrimination, cannot be 'legitimated or justified as medical necessity.'

Psychiatric bodies accept that medical necessity is insufficient alone to 'justify involuntary treatment of capable persons.' However, it is essential to ensure that involuntary treatment is used only when it is appropriate, and other interventions are unlikely to succeed (Lieberman, Levin and Ruiz, 2013).

The criticism that solitary confinement and restraint may constitute torture

Méndez (2013, paragraph 63) rejects a therapeutic justification for solitary confinement and sustained restraint of disabled people psychiatric settings. Both interventions may constitute torture and ill-treatment. An 'absolute ban' on these and other coercive, non-consensual interventions should apply in 'psychiatric and social care institutions.' Using restraint and seclusion can lead to further non-consensual treatment like forced medication and ECT (Méndez, 2013, paragraph 63).

Lieberman, Levin and Ruiz (2013) state that for psychotic patients trying to severely injure themselves or others, restraint may be the 'only way to prevent severe injury' to the patient and protect others. They note that restrained patients must be monitored carefully, and restraints should be for the shortest time possible.

The criticism that guardianship should not allow justification of forced treatment

Méndez (2013, paragraph 65) is concerned that having been 'stripped' of their legal capacity, people with disabilities may be appointed a guardian or someone else that can make their decisions. The consent of these representative will be considered enough to 'justify forced treatment.'

For Lieberman, Levin and Ruiz (2013) an appropriate determination that someone lacks ability to make their own decisions, and which is reached to protect their rights, ought to be 'commended and not condemned.'

The view that institutionalising legislation should be abolished

Méndez (2013, paragraph 68) calls for abolishing laws which authorise institutionalising disabled people because of their disability 'without their free and informed consent.' This includes instances where the grounds of 'care, treatment and public security' are legally linked to mental disorder.

Opposing all this, Lieberman, Levin and Ruiz (2013) say that hospitalisation of people with psychiatric disorders can be life-saving. It can lead to the person having restored to them the 'ability to direct his or her own life.'

The criticism that severity of mental illness should not justify deprivation of liberty

For Méndez (2013, paragraph 69) depriving liberty owing to mental illness is unjustified if based on discrimination or prejudice against disabled people. The severity of the mental disorder is not by itself enough to 'justify detention' and such detention must be needed to 'protect the safety of the person or of others.' Except in emergency, someone should not be deprived of liberty unless they are of unsound mind. Detention in a psychiatric context may lead to non-consensual psychiatric treatment. Therefore, depriving someone of their liberty on the grounds of a disability, and where it causes 'severe pain or suffering' could come under the remit of *Convention against Torture*.

Lieberman, Levin and Ruiz (2013) argue that the severe impairment and suffering because of mental illness 'can be an appropriate basis for involuntary hospitalization.'

Other criticisms

Criticism referring misleadingly to a genetic 'basis' of schizophrenia

Orthodox practitioners tend to reject that genes are solely a direct cause of schizophrenia. Genetics' role in increasing susceptibility to schizophrenia may relate to 'specific environmental factors' (Torrey, 2019, p. 131). Genes may play a 'modest' role with schizophrenia not being 'primarily a genetic disease' (Ibid., p. 133). Also, genetic, lifestyle, and environmental factors interact (National Library of Medicine, 2021).

According to dissenters 'mainstream psychiatry' mistakenly accepts 'the genetic **basis** of schizophrenia' and the condition being 'a **genetically based** disorder' (Joseph, 2013, pp. 83 and 85, bold added). Rose (2019) rejects that we have discovered 'anything about the genetic **basis**' of schizophrenia (Ibid. p. 107, bold added).

But such criticisms avoid explaining the phrase 'genetic basis.' It may mean that genetic factors act exclusively without the complex interaction of other factors, or that genes are foundational and more important than lifestyle or environmental influences. Any such implied centrality would not reflect an orthodox view, blunting the criticism.

Criticising nebulous targets

Sometimes the target of criticisms about genetic theories is unclear. It said that 'mainstream psychiatry' sees the genetic basis of schizophrenia as a proven fact; that 'psychiatry' has uncritically accepted the conclusions of schizophrenia twin and adoption researchers; and that 'the discipline' has failed to critically analyse its own research (Joseph, 2013, p. 85).

These are vague targets, and as a result, people's understanding of them is likely to vary. It is unclear whom you question when you want to know what 'psychiatry' is saying. Criticism would be more plausible if directed towards individuals who could then confirm or deny what they believed was a 'proven fact.' Otherwise, criticism becomes targetless and therefore pointless.

Similarly, where dissenters mention eugenics, forced sterilisation, and mass murder, the broad and vague expression 'biological psychiatry' is used to draw a parallel between Nazi psychiatrists and modern-day psychiatrists (Read and Masson, 2013a).

Imputed (sometimes malign) motivations in genetic research

Critics may maintain that genetic theories help the interests of social and political elites, and the pharmaceutical business. They allow these entities to claim that 'psychological distress' has a physical cause rather than being brought about by the family, social, and political setting (Joseph, 2013, p. 85). But such accusations of motives towards unnamed researchers, are too vague. Dissenters might more precisely and more convincingly argue for more attention to be paid to family, social, and political factors relating to schizophrenia.

In a more sinister vein, in a book chapter, 'Genetics, Eugenics, and the Mass Murder of Schizophrenics,' Read and Masson (2013) discuss Nazi atrocities. Genetic theories it is said gave to what happened the 'motivation, the rationale, and the camouflage.' Psychiatrists helped develop the theory 'that undesirable behaviour is genetically transmitted' used to justify 'compulsory sterilisation and mass murder.' These theories 'still dominate psychiatry today' (Ibid., p. 34). Mental health workers should remain alert to their own 'failures to perceive' the ways in which people are harmed by others including, 'by mental health workers themselves' (Ibid., p. 43).

The implication seems to be that genetic researchers today would want to justify compulsory sterilisation and mass murder. Most notably, the authors fail to name a single modern-day researcher that they might be talking about.

The criticism that after the failed dopamine hypothesis, researchers considered other neurochemicals

Critics have stated that the 'continued failure to confirm biological psychiatry's lead hypothesis led to the investigation of other neurotransmitters' (Read, 2013a, p. 66). If it is accepted that confirmation of the dopamine hypothesis did not 'fail,' but pointed to refinements, it is misleading to suggest that this 'led to' researchers turning to other neurotransmitters. In fact, the dopamine hypothesis continued and continues to be developed.

Research into other neurotransmitters also continues including their interaction with dopamine. In examining the role of dopamine in schizophrenia, Brisch and colleagues (2014) note that, to the present day, 'the mechanism of every effective antipsychotic medication in schizophrenia involves dopamine and its interaction with other neurochemical pathways such as those of glutamate, GABA, serotonin, and acetylcholine' (Ibid.).

ECT historical cases conflated with modern findings

Historically, according to Read, Mosher and Bentall (2013, pp. 96–97), psychiatrists supporting ECT considered damaging the brain beneficial. Freeman (1941, p. 83) stated, 'The greater the damage, the more likely the remission of psychotic symptoms.' Myerson (1942) said, 'Some of the very best cures that one gets are in those individuals whom one reduces almost to amentia.' Supposedly continuing the same theme, Perrin et al. (2012) found the ECT reduces the brain's 'functional connectivity' correcting a supposed, 'hyperconnectivity' in depressed people. Are Read, Mosher and Bentall (2013, pp. 96–97) saying that Perrin sees 'brain damage' as beneficial? Surely this could be made clearer.

References

Baghramian, M. (2001) 'Relativism: Philosophical aspects' *International Encyclopaedia of Social and Behavioural Sciences.* London, Elsevier.

Bracken, P., Thomas, P., Timimi, S., Asen, E., Behr, G., Beuster, C., Bhunnoo, S. and colleagues (2012) 'Psychiatry beyond the current paradigm' *British Journal of Psychiatry* 201, 430–434. https://pubmed.ncbi.nlm.nih.gov/23209088/

Brandon, P., Cowley, C., McDonald, P., Neville, R., Palmer, S., Wellstood-Easonandon, S. (1985) 'Leicester ECT trial' *British Journal of Psychiatry* 146, 177–183.

Brisch, R., Saniotis, A., Wolf, R., Bielau, H., Bernstein, H.-G., Steiner, J., Bogerts, B., Braun, K., Jankowski, Z., Kumaratilake, J., Henneberg, M. and Gos, T. (2014) 'The role of dopamine in schizophrenia from a neurobiological and evolutionary perspective: Old fashioned, but still in vogue' *Frontiers in Psychiatry* (19 May 2014). https://www.ncbi.nlm.nih.gov/pmc/articles/PMC4032934/

Campbell, P. (2010) 'Surviving the system' in Basset, T. and Stickley, T. (Eds.) *Voices of Experience: Narratives of Mental Health Survivors.* Chichester, Wiley-Blackwell.

Cardno, A. G. and Gottesman, I. I. (2000). 'Twin studies of schizophrenia: From bow-and-arrow concordances to star wars Mx and functional genomics' *American Journal of Medical Genetics* 97, 12–17. https://pubmed.ncbi.nlm.nih.gov/10813800/

Cooke, A. (Ed.) (2017) *Understanding Psychosis and Schizophrenia: Why people sometimes hear voices, believe things that others find strange, or appear out of touch with reality, and what can help.* British Psychological Society Division of Clinical Psychology/Canterbury Christchurch University.

Davies, J. (2014) *Cracked: Why Psychiatry Is Doing More Harm than Good.* London, Icon Books.

Freeman, W. (1941) 'Brain damaging therapeutics' *Diseases of the Nervous System* 2, 83.

Freeman, C. and Kendall, R. (1980) 'ECT: patients' experiences and attitudes' *British Journal of Psychiatry* 137, 8–16. https://www.cambridge.org/core/journals/the-british-journal-of-psychiatry/article/abs/ect-i-patients-experiences-and-attitudes/5EA1482773BCD3AE8EC295D6B133B418

Granholm, E. and Loh, K. (2009) 'Evidence-based psychosocial interventions for schizophrenia' Kasper, S. and Papadimitriou, G. N. (Eds.) (2009) (2nd. Edition) *Schizophrenia: Biopsychosocial Approaches and Current Challenges* (Medical Psychiatry Series). New York and London, Informa Healthcare (pp. 269–281).

Griffiths, C. and O'Niell-Kerr (2019) 'Patients', carers', and the public's perspectives on electroconvulsive therapy' *Frontiers of Psychiatry* 10, 304. www.ncbi.nlm.nih.gov/pmc/articles/PMC6514218/

Hamilton, M. (1960) 'A rating scale for depression' *Journal of Neurology, Neurosurgery and Psychiatry* 23, 1, 56–62 (February). https://pubmed.ncbi.nlm.nih.gov/14399272/

Henriksen, M. G., Nordgaard, J. and Jansson, L. B. (2017) 'Genetics of schizophrenia: Overview of methods, findings and limitations' *Frontiers of Human Neuroscience* 11, 322. https://research.regionh.dk/files/68915239/Henriksen_MG_Nordgaard_J_Jansson_LB_Genetics_2017.pdf

Howes, O. D. and Kapur, S. (2009) 'The dopamine hypothesis of schizophrenia: Version III—the final common pathway' *Schizophrenia Bulletin* 35, 3, 549–562. https://pubmed.ncbi.nlm.nih.gov/19325164/

Hutton, P., Weinmann, S., Bola, J. and Read, R. (2013) 'Antipsychotic drugs' in Read, J. and Dillon, J. (Eds.) (2nd Edition) *Models of Madness: Psychological, Social and Biological Approaches to Psychosis*. London and New York, Routledge (pp. 105–124).

Jauhar, S., Nour, M. M., Verones, M., Rogdaki, M., Bonoldi, I., Azis, M., Turkheimer, F., McGuire, P., Young, A. H. and Howes, O. D. (2017) 'A test of the transdiagnostic dopamine hypothesis of psychosis using positron emission tomographic imaging in bipolar affective disorder and schizophrenia' *JAMA Psychiatry* 74, 12, 1206–1213 (December). https://www.semanticscholar.org/paper/A-Test-of-the-Transdiagnostic-Dopamine-Hypothesis-Jauhar-Nour/aadbe9adb12a2a7131f1ce78f58025a5dc4abd2c

Johnstone, E. C., Deakin, J. F. W., Lawler, P., Frith, C. D., Stevens, M. and McPherson, K. (1980) 'The Northwick Park electroconvulsive therapy trial' *Lancet* 2, 1317–1320. https://pubmed.ncbi.nlm.nih.gov/6109147/

Joseph, J. (2013) '"Schizophrenia" and heredity: Why the emperor (still) has no genes' in Read, J. and Dillon, J. (2013) (2nd Edition) *Models of Madness: Psychological, Social and Biological Approaches to Psychosis*. London and New York, Routledge (pp. 72–89).

Joseph, J. (2023) *Schizophrenia and Genetics: The End of an Illusion*. New York and London, Routledge.

Levin, A. (2014) 'UN report says common psychiatric practices amount to "torture"' *Psychiatric News* (American Psychiatric Association 25 April 2014). https://psychnews.psychiatryonline.org/doi/full/10.1176/appi.pn.2014.5a11

Lieberman, J., Levin, S. and Ruiz, P. (2013) 'Joint statement from the American Psychiatric Association and the World Psychiatric Association' in Center for Human Rights and Humanitarian Law: Anti-Torture Initiative (2013) *Torture in Healthcare Settings: Reflections on the Special Report on Torture's 2013 Thematic Report*. American University Washington College of Law – Center for Human Rights and Humanitarian Law (December 2013) (pp. 141–146).

Méndez, J. E. (2013) *Report of the Special Rapporteur on Torture and Other Cruel, Inhuman or Degrading Treatment or Punishment*. New York, United Nations, Human Rights Council. http://www.hr-dp.org/files/2013/10/28/A.HRC.22.53SpecialRappReport.2013.pdf

Myerson, A. (1942) 'Fatalities following ECT' *Transactions of the American Neurological Association* 68, 39.

National Library of Medicine (2021) 'What does it mean to have a genetic predisposition to a disease?' *National Library of Medicine* (Bethesda, Maryland, May 2021). https://medlineplus.gov/genetics/understanding/mutationsanddisorders/predisposition/

NHS (reviewed November, 2019) *Schizophrenia Causes*. https://www.nhs.uk/mental-health/conditions/schizophrenia/causes/

NICE (2003, 2009, 2014) *Guidance on the use of electroconvulsive therapy: Technology appraisal guidance TA 59* (Published 2003, Updated 2009, Static list review 2014). www.nice.org.uk/guidance/ta59

Perrin, J. S., Merz, S., Bennett, D. M., Currie, J., Steele, D. J., Reid, I. C. and Schwartzbauer, C. (2012) 'Electro convulsive therapy reduces frontal cortical connectivity in severe depressive disorder' *Biological Sciences* 109, 14, 5464–5468 (March 19 2012). 10.1073/pnas.1117206109

Petrides, G. and Braga, R. J. (2009) 'Electroconvulsive therapy in schizophrenia' in Kasper, S. and Papadimitriou, G. N. (Eds.) (2nd Edition) *Schizophrenia: Biopsychosocial Approaches and Current Challenges* (Medical Psychiatry Series). New York and London, Informa Healthcare (pp. 290–298).

Read, J. (2013a) 'Biological psychiatry's lost cause: The schizophrenic brain' in Read, J. and Dillon, J. (Eds.) (2nd Edition) *Models of Madness: Psychological, Social and Biological Approaches to Psychosis*. London and New York, Routledge (pp. 62–71).

Read, J., Haslam, N. and Magliano, L. (2013) 'Prejudice, stigma and "schizophrenia": The role of bio-genetic ideology' in Read, J. and Dillon, J. (Eds.) (2nd Edition) *Models of Madness: Psychological, Social and Biological Approaches to Psychosis*. London and New York, Routledge (pp. 157–177).

Read, J. and Masson, J. (2013) 'Genetics, eugenics, and the mass murder of "schizophrenics"' in Read, J. and Dillon, J. (Eds.) (2nd Edition) *Models of Madness: Psychological, Social and Biological Approaches to Psychosis*. London and New York, Routledge (pp. 34–46).

Read, J., Mosher, L. and Bentall, R. (2013) 'Schizophrenia is not an illness' in Read, J. and Dillon, J. (Eds.) (2nd Edition) *Models of Madness: Psychological, Social and Biological Approaches to Psychosis*. London and New York, Routledge (pp. 3–8).

Read, J., Bentall, R., Johnstone, L., Fosse, R. and Bracken, P. (2013) 'Electroconvulsive therapy' in Read, J. and Dillon, J. (Eds.) (2nd Edition) *Models of Madness: Psychological, Social and Biological Approaches to Psychosis*. London and New York, Routledge (pp. 92).

Rose, N. (2019) *Our Psychiatric Future: The Politics of Mental Health*. Medford, Mass, Polity Press.

Schosser, A. and McGuffin, P. (2009) 'Genetic and epigenetic factors in schizophrenia' in Kasper, S. and Papadimitriou, G. N. (Eds.) (2nd Edition) *Schizophrenia: Biopsychosocial Approaches and Current Challenges* (Medical Psychiatry Series). New York and London, Informa Healthcare.

Selten, J-P., van der Ven, E., Rutten, B. and Cantor-Graae, E. (2013) 'The social defeat hypothesis of schizophrenia: An update' *Schizophrenia Bulletin* 39, 6, 1180–1186 (November). https://pubmed.ncbi.nlm.nih.gov/24062592/

Sullivan, P. F., Kendler, K. S. and Neale, M. C. (2003) 'Schizophrenia as a complex trait: Evidence from a meta-analysis of twin studies' *Archives of General Psychiatry* 60, 1187–1192. https://pubmed.ncbi.nlm.nih.gov/14662550/

Taylor, P. and Fleminger, J. (1980) 'ECT for schizophrenia' *Lancet* 1, 380.

Torrey, E. F. (2019) (7th Edition) *Surviving Schizophrenia: A Family Manual*. New York and London, Harper Perennial.

INDEX

abnormal neural activity 75
Abraham, K. 125
acetylcholine 92–93
ACT *see* assertive community
    treatment (ACT)
Aderhold, V. 79, 153
Alem, A. 114, 159
American Psychiatric Association 127
amphetamines 34
Andreasen, N. 83, 84, 156
antibiotics 115
antipsychotics 13, 104–105; action of
    107; adverse effects of 112–113;
    antibiotics 115; chlorpromazine
    106, 116; critics
    misrepresenting an orthodox
    position about 157; dissenting
    views and weaknesses 112;
    failed neurochemical
    explanations and 168; Faustian
    descriptions of sedation 115;
    first-generation, action of 108;
    movement disorders 110;
    orthodox and dissenting
    positions 105; research and
    claims associated with
    pharmaceutical companies
    111–112; schizophrenia in
    developing countries 113–115;
    second-generation, action of

108–109; sedation 110, 115;
    sexual side effects 110–111; side
    effects of 109–111; types and
    efficacy 106–107; weight
    gain 109
Appelbaum, P. S. 139, 170
assertive community treatment (ACT)
    133, 135–136, 144
AstraZeneca 150
Avramopoulos, D. 62

*Bad Pharma: How Drug Companies
    Mislead Doctors and Harm
    Patients* 111
Baron, M. 63
Bentall, R. 22, 23, 26, 40, 41, 151, 154,
    155, 165, 174
Bini, L. 124
bio-genetic ideology 167
bio-genetic psychiatry 53
biological markers 60
biological psychiatry 45, 84, 90, 98
biopsychosocial perspective of
    schizophrenia 11, 31–32;
    criticisms 40–41; family therapy
    35; identification and diagnosis
    33; illness, schizophrenia as an
    39–40; language of criticism 41,
    42; medical condition 32–33;
    medical model 36–38, 42;